I0421179

For Lynda,

Who found that the greatest learning about yourself happens at the most painful times.

Foolish the doctor who despises

knowledge acquired by the ancients.

- Hippocrates

Preface

Often my books take the reader on a magic carpet to an ancient world or perhaps in a time machine to a future place where possible research might live. In this book it is not so. To experience the true nature of Basil a different type of quietness is required. Here, we must journey to the centre of the Earth, to the hottest place imaginable. It is dark and lonely.

As you pass through the doorway of the mountain, you reach a clearing where the sun shines bright and hot. It is a tiny space and all around you are doorways to take you deeper into the darkness. In the centre of the chasm is a crystal blue lake; the light glints on the water and shoots rainbow droplets from the waterfall above.

By the side of the lake, in this burning shadeless sun, a peppery leaf grows with zesty green leaves. Across the ripples, her fragrance drifts. And through the rustle of the leaves you think perhaps...you might have heard.... a whisper...some kind of imperceptible clue.

But to what? You *cannot* be sure.

It is nothing more than a feeling, an instinct, perhaps even less.

Because, if there is a sensation that you dare not even put into words....then I would suggest to you that Basil has probably spoken. A discrete whisper, no more. A breeze so light it only just moves the leaves.

Smile in the plant's direction, but if you take my advice you'll stay this side of the water. For she..... is not a plant to be messed with. No need to touch her, simply inhale the vapours she emits. For she can prepare you for any pain you might encounter and on Basil's journey, I can promise you, you will.

Look around you. There are many entrances into the mountain to lead you to the chasm below. There is no turning back. You must continue onward for no healing can begin without this pilgrimage underground.

But choices seem much simpler now.

You sense you can safely enter any doorway you choose. Relish the new sense of bravery about what lies ahead. You have absorbed the incredible power of the Basil plant.

Introduction

When you enter into Basil's world, you go through a gateway into a very strange world, of misdirection, of disagreements and the last straw snapping. When Basil comes into play, anything that has been outgrown or no longer serves the soul pathway will be kicked into touch.

This is a bravery book. The courage it has taken me to write it (and it has been harder than any of the books I have written so far) and the fortitude of the patient to face demons he feared he could not look in the eye.

On Amazon I describe myself as "less Titania, more Gimli son of Gloin" as a testament not only to my short, fat, hairy legs, ginger beard and grumpy demeanour, but also the fact that I have never been afraid of travelling underground with my medicine. The deeper the emotional trauma, the harder I swing the pick axe, because like any dwarf, I know that the deeper you go the more likely it is that things will glint and sparkle and treasures will be found.

There are, though, some doors in the mountain inside my head that even I wouldn't want to open. Who knows what monsters lay behind *them*? They're the ones connected to failure, defeat and times when my self esteem was mortally wounded, and I left it there to die. The stench of its decomposition emanates through, stinging my bodymind, but I dare not look its way. Instead I paint on a lipstick smile and find a distraction to avert my gaze. Still though, I sense the aching wail from beyond the chasm.

When I started to research Sweet Basil, I had no idea of the journey I would be taken on. I wouldn't have chosen it if I had. I hadn't sharpened my axe and no sword would have been strong enough to slay the dragons I knew lay inwait.

And yet...

Here I still am

After facing some of the worst things about myself over the last couple of months, I find I am smiling so much more! Questions have been contemplated and answered and, admittedly I do feel like I have gone through seven rounds against a flail but I feel on top of the world. I literally feel lighter because of it.

In this book the physical medicine isn't that interesting, I don't think. It is the spiritual and emotional aspects that are so fascinating. Because of that, this book is upside down! The physical medicine comes at the end and the emotional, spiritual and magical parts at the front.

Come with me, into the chamber, you'll need a flashlight down here. (I'm brave enough to open the door and lead you in now, if you notice) And one last question before we enter...

How do you feel about scorpions?

Table of Contents

Chapter 1- The History of Basil

From a researcher's point of view, the amount of historical information available about uses and symbolism of Sweet Basil is staggering. That *should* mean it is very easy to get to the heart of the plant. But at every possible turning, you will find there are contradictions, arguments and disagreements. The strange thing is, the more I have studied, the more I find that every viewpoint is correct.

The effects of Basil are wholly dependent on the patient it is used upon. More than any other plant, Basil affects every person differently.

Ethnobotany always starts by looking at the place a plant grows and the environment it lives in. Now, normally that pertains to the soil, what it lives next to, what climate it is has to deal with. All of these add to the chemistry of the plant. Of course, here that will still be so, but as you'll see there seems to be more than that at play.

In 1653 Nicholas Culpepper wrote in his Complete Herbal...

This is the herb which all authors are together by the ears about, and rail at one another (like lawyers). Galen and Dioscorides hold it not fitting to be taken inwardly; and Chrysippus rails at it with downright Billingsgate rhetoric; Pliny, and the Arabian physicians, defend it.

For my own part, I presently found that speech true:

Non nostrum inter nos tantas componere lites.

[Translates to: I am not the one to conclude this argument]

And away to Dr. Reason went I, who told me it was an herb of Mars, and under the scorpion, and, perhaps therefore called Basilican, and it is no marvel if it carry a kind of virulent quality with it. Being applied to the place bitten by venomous beasts, or stung by a wasp or hornet, it speedily draws the poison to it. Every like draws his like. Mizaldus affirms, that being laid to rot in horse-dung, it will breed venomous beasts. Hilarius, a French physician, affirms upon his own knowledge, that an acquaintance of his, by common smelling to it, had a scorpion bred in his brain. Something is the matter this herb and rue will not grow together, no, nor near one another; and we know rue is as great an enemy to poison as any that grows.

To conclude: It expelleth both birth and after-birth; and as it helps the deficiency of Venus in one kind, so it spoils all her actions in another. I dare write no more of it.

I dare write no more of it. *Dare...*

14

Now, one might wonder what it is that worries him so much. Is it the decision about whether one should ingest Basil or not? (In 400 years we don't seem to have come that far do we? This is the argument still echoing through every Facebook page!) Or does he feel concern about the *plant?* For as he points out, the rue plant is very discriminating about where it grows. It won't thrive where it finds anything poisonous. Does *Rue* worry about Basil too?

Well, actually as you review much of the ancient literature about this bright green herb, there is a resounding theme that runs through them. Scorpions breed under pots of Basil, they say. If you sniff Basil then scorpions breed inside your head. If you bang two Basil leaves together, scorpions will appear. If you chew Basil leaves and spit them out, *worms* will appear. It's rare that anyone has anything nice to say about Basil.

This might have arisen from its name.

Ocimum Basilicum

The name Basil comes from the word Basileus which means "king" in Greek and so it might be referring to the plant fit for a king. Some sources suggest it might attest to Basil being included in some royal anointing oil, but I cannot find any evidence to sustain that claim. The *Basilisk* is the name of the medieval creature that would fix you with its stare and turn you to stone. The best representation of the Basilisk is found in heraldry where the Basilisk is usually depicted with the head and legs of a cock, a snake-like tail, and a body like a bird's. Sometimes wings are shown as being covered with feathers but the really fearsome pictures show the creature as covered in scales. Perhaps this is the first attribution of the plant to serpents and dragons.

Interestingly, the Romans referred to the terrifying Basilisk as *"regulus"* which also means "Little King." The name refers, not to the crown that sometimes we see on its head, but more the manner in which he terrorises other creatures with his violent stare.

So, where did it come from, this peppery, hot herb? In truth it is not really known for certain, but common opinion says it probably came from Africa and Asia and was bought to Europe by Alexander the Great in the 4th Century BC. It is first recorded in England in the 1500s and in the US in the 1600s.

Today, Basil is used in cookery across the globe, most notably in Italy, Thailand and Greece. I say notably about

Greece because to the *Ancient* Greeks it was unheard of to eat such a thing. To consume the energies of Basil would have been mocking the fates and a ludicrous and dangerous thing to do. It was considered sacred. Just as they still do today, they considered that it would ward off evil and was a deterrent to mosquitoes (which it is!), but in the days of a deeper philosophy, their beliefs ran deeper. The connection seemed, somehow, to do with death and a love eternal. It came to signify mourning and would be placed on the graves of loved ones.

The Greeks spoke of how Basil had originated in honour of Ocimus, the great man who had organized the combats staged in honour of Pallas. Pallas, it is said had ruled Paralia or perhaps Diacria. A fearsome man of the greatest virility (he fathered 50 sons) Ocimus was killed by a gladiator. Legend has it that where he fell, Basil appeared.

In Greece, and in Rome, Basil suffered a terrible reputation associated with poverty, hate and misfortune. This was mainly down to the belief that Basil would only prosper if showered with abuse. It became customary to shout and curse when sowing Basil seeds in an effort to make them thrive in this hostile environment. Later this led to the

French phrase, still in general use today, *'semer le Basilic'* *"sow the Basil"* or to slander someone.

"The emblem of the Devil!" they believed in Crete and because of this it was placed on window ledges to protect against his entry into the house.

Basil charms the Devil.

Grown in many medieval gardens, Basil is mentioned by several early writers. A very early historical reference comes from Chrysippus of Cnidos, a Greek philosopher of note from the 4th century BC. Culpepper's right, he really does rail! He declares Basil capable of harming the liver, weakening the eyes, causing madness and damaging the liver. This is, he says, why even goats will not touch the herb.

By contrast, Philistion of Locri (philosopher - 4th century) and Plistonicus (physician 3rd-4th centuries) both attest that Basil would be the choice of herb to use **on patients who had lost vitality.** This is very interesting to me because Philistion was Chrisippus's tutor. So somehow they have differed to each other in thinking over this herb. Both Galen and Dioscorides seem to err on the side of caution too, and neither advocate taking Basil internally, which is unusual for either of them.

Dioscorides has much more to say about Basil. He describes how he uses it for:

- Dimness of sight and rheums of the eyes
- To provoke sneezing
- That the oil is warming and used in the vulva is emmenogogue and abortifacient
- Bites from sea dragons and scorpion stings
- Toothache (leaves pounded into oil)
- Mad dog
- Viper bites
- The seed taken in drink corrects excess of black bile
- Difficulty of urination (through a diuretic action)
- Flatulence
- Encourage breast milk
- Softens stools for easier passing
- Dandruff

He also relates how he knows that African people, living close to habitats of large numbers of scorpions, eat Basil and then know they will be without pain when they are stung. Can you visualise the stories passing from merchant to merchant as the camels cross the many miles of sands, then being passed to him in his Roman market in a tempt to get him to buy their aromatic wares?

John Gerard was a very well respected herbalist and writer of the 16th century. He was a barber-surgeon who maintained an enormous herbal garden in London. He would have been one of the main herbal dispensers of the period. A controversial figure amongst other naturalists of the time, he was a doer, not a thinker, and his ardour to put his theories into practice made him somewhat of an outsider in the trendy naturalist society of Lime Street at the time.

Nevertheless, Gerard set about writing *The Herbal or Generall History of Plants*. This was a stunningly beautiful work with gorgeous botanical drawings and the deliciously florid language Gerard liked to use. Actually, most of the work was plagiarised from an earlier book by Dutchman, Rembert Dodoens, and a herbal he had written in 1554. Gerard had simply added some plants from his garden and also some new ones that had recently been brought back from the Americas.

Potentially, if it wasn't for the sheer beauty of the book, it might not have survived history because much of the information contained has subsequently been proven to be wrong, but his writings on Basil seem to echo many of those from the time. *Melancholy, headaches and snake bites,* we will see this over and over again. Incidentally, this is probably a timely point for a reminder that essential oils were not in general usage yet (although they were being made in some large houses with still rooms) and the herbals of this period discuss decoctions, infusions and the like.

He claimed that Basil juice, *"drunke in wine of Chios or strong Sacke,"* cures headaches. *Mixed with barley meal, rose oil, and vinegar, Basil juice was also used as an anti-inflammatory and as an antidote for snakebites. According to Gerard, "the seed drunke is a remedy for melancholy people; for those that are short-winded, and them that can hardly make water."*

John Parkinson was a founder member of the Worshipful Society of Apothecaries. Owner of a beautiful botanical garden in Long Acre, Covent Garden (which would be just round the corner from Trafalgar Square on today's maps), Parkinson was to rise to the elite position of Apothecary to King Charles I. When in 1617 he became a member of the Society of Aporthecaries, he served on a committee that was to create one of the most important medicinal documents we have today. The *Pharmacopœia Londinensis* or London Pharmacy was a complete and detailed list of all plants that every apothecary of the period should stock.

Later, in the service of the king, he was to write two exquisite works. The first came about after having spent time with the new young queen, Henrietta I. Arriving in England from France at the tender age of 15, she was understandably nervous and craving something to occupy her mind. Parkinson came to her rescue, escorting her on daily forays into the garden, strolling through the flowerbeds, and teaching her the ways of the plants. From their time together a book grew, published in 1629, Paradisi in Sole Paradisus Terrestris (*Park-in-Sun's Terrestrial Paradise*) You'll notice Parkinson's little play on his name in the title.

But the most glorious description, I feel, is found in the subtitle he gave his work: *A Garden of all sorts of pleasant flowers which our English ayre will permit to be noursed up.* The book, which he described as his "Speaking Garden" was dedicated to the queen.

Then in 1640, he took up his quill again, this time creating *Theatrum Botanicum* (*The Botanical Theatre* or *Theatre of Plants*). This was to become the masterpiece that we best remember him for today. It is probably the most complete picture of plants used in medicine in the 17th century. As well as being extensive, it is breathtakingly exquisitely illustrated and very witty too.

In *Theatrum Botanicum* he describes how Basil has a "scent fit for the house of a king." Appropriate wording coming from someone who works for the monarch, but also, of course, about a plant with a Latin name such as Basilicum.

He tells us to

- Mix with honey to take away ulcers and that it also eases spots.
- Add to goose grease for children's earache
- Use to procure a "cheerful and merry heart"
- It comforts the heart and trembling thereof
- Mix with rose and vinegar to help those with dropsy, jaundice and lethargy

(For those not fluent in medieval disease...dropsy is what we would now describe as oedema, swelling or fluid retention)

And wait for it

"It provoketh the venery so is oft given to horses to help them to breed"

Venery? Dictionary please

venery[1]

ˈvɛn(ə)ri/

noun

archaic

Sexual indulgence.

"Not a few of them engaged in venery"

Ooo...I say! Now tell me you haven't got visions you'd rather not have....with or without horses! (Now you've *definitely* got horses haven't you?!)

Helpfully, he was also able to disclose that Arabian authors recommend it for **melancholy and sadness that seems to manifest for no reason.**

And then he tells a fascinating tale that will colour the tone of my book throughout.

Franciscus Farchis, Advocate of the State of Genoa went on an ambassadorial visit to the Duke of Milan and with him, he took a sprig of Basil. The Duke looked at him quizzically and asked him what it meant. Farchis smiled and said "Basil had a lovely smell if gently handled, but if hardly wrung would breed scorpions" The Duke was pleased with the witty answer and sent him away honourably.

But, reading his phrase, there is no doubting there a sense of underlying threat, is there? Treat us nicely or you'll be sorry. (I also remember that we are told to rip Basil, not chop it, aren't we? Is that handling it more gently do we think?)

And when you dig deeper, you find there is this dual symbolism reverberating through historical references. Love – Hate, Peace-War, Life and Death.

In Italy, but also in Greece and Romania in particular Basil symbolises love. Sprigs are given as love tokens and in some parts of the country it is customary for a woman to put a pot of Basil on her balcony if she is ready for courtship. In others, a suitor would wear a sprig in his hat and then the lady could look through her window and decide whether to pursue the romance or to have him sent away. (How much easier would courtship be, if we still used these symbolisms? I am not sure we have progressed you know!!!)

So where did this strange anachronism originate? How did Basil go from being the herb of the Devil, associated with poverty and hatred to evolving to take on the mantle of love? Is it a reflection of our present day wedding vows "for richer, for poorer, in sickness and in health..."?

One possible suggestion might come from the connection of Basil with the Greek Orthodox Church. Helena, the mother of Constantine the Great went on a pilgrimage to the Holy Land in 326AD. Legend has it that she came upon a field, filled with a strange and beauteous smelling herb, such as she had never seen the like. The herb, she was told, was called Valsiliko, since the word Basileus means of the king.

Beneath the growing Basil, were found three crosses and amongst them a sign, inscribed "Jesus of Nazareth, the King of the Jews". But how to know which had belonged to The Christ, and which had crucified the thieves with whom he had been died, she wondered? Helena, now a very sick and frail woman of 80 years, was told to kiss each of the crosses. She did so, and when she kissed the third cross, a great miracle was seen as Helena was made entirely well.

It just so happened, that at that time, a funeral procession was passing by. Helena approached the party and begged them to lay their dead body onto the cross. The man was brought back to life, which is now why The One True Cross is also known as The Life Giving Cross. Of course, it is believed that the cross giveth life to all who believeth in Him.

When the True Cross was identified, it was lifted on high for everyone to see. The crowd sang *Kyrie eleison* for many hours. This practice is still enacted at current celebrations of The One True Cross which is held on September 14th in Greek Orthodox Churches around the world. The devotional altar of the service is filled with Basil in memory of that day.

Here, we can clearly see attributions of life and death. Even love conquering all, but where did all these *darker* attributions come from?

Common thinking agrees it might have arisen from a 14th Century story written by Boccaccio in a series of tales called the Decameron. The author relates how in Messina (Italy) there lived three merchant brothers and their sister, Isabetta. Radiant, as she was, soon she captivated the eye of a young man in their employ, Lorenzo.

The two began to court secretly and fell deeply in love. The brothers of course, as brothers do, found out and were consumed with worry for Isabetta's reputation. They hatched a plan.

Asking Lorenzo if he would join them in a meeting, they lured him outside of the city walls. There they killed and buried him in a shallow grave. Deepening their deception, they lied to Isabetta on their return, concocting a tale of how Lorenzo had been called away on business.

That night, as Isabetta slept, a terrifying dream befell her. Lorenzo appeared at her bed and disclosed the horrifying truth of his death. Describing the murder in detail he whispered the secret location of his grave. Isabetta flew from her city in her nightclothes, There, just as Lorenzo had told her, she uncovered the body of her love with her bare hands. Distraught, Isabetta frantically tried to think of a way to keep Lorenzo with her, but she knew she could not salvage all of his remains alone. Taking her knife, she cut off his head, hid it under her night gown and silently returned home.

Isabetta was terrified her brothers might uncover her secret and knew she had to hide the severed head. Burying it into a pot, she planted some Basil on top. Retreating to her room, Isabella locked herself in.

For months, Isabetta wept for her love. She would sit, clenching the pot tightly to her and as she cried, her tears fell into the Basil pot. Nourished by her pain the plant grew strong and healthy and with it so did her obsession.

As days turned to weeks, and then weeks to months, the brothers became suspicious of Isabetta's strange attachment to the Basil. Knowing best, as brothers do, they took the plant away from her. They confiscated it and uprooted the plant to throw it away. As the roots lifted from the soil, her grim discovery was revealed as Lorenzo's lifeless eyes stared back at them. Knowing they had been discovered the brothers fled the city. Isabetta separated yet again from her love, died of a broken heart.

To my mind, I have another suspicion that another far older story might have triggered the tale. Some say that when Salome presented the head of John the Baptist on a plate, it was garnished with fragrant leaves of basil! His diabolical demise sanctioned by Salome's mother Herodias, when her maniacal rage at The Baptist after he had declared her second marriage unlawful, became a very unholy preoccupation.

Love...but not healthy love. Obsessive, jealous and cruel love. All consuming, secretive and dangerous love. It reminds me of that Harry Warren song "I only have eyes for you..." I remember, as a fresh faced ingénue practicing ballet to the Art Garfunkel version and thinking it was the most romantic thing I had ever heard. Now as a grown woman, I find its intensity disturbing and vaguely unnatural. As I pass from maiden, to mother and soon to crone...there's no way I'd want that for my child. But how on earth does one convey that truth. *Hold that thought....*

Chapter 2 - The Spiritual Dimensions of Basil

Archetype

Ezulie

Ezulie is voodoo Loa, or goddess, she stands for love, beauty and passion. She is a triple goddess and offerings to her are made in the form of Basil. To me, here, encapsulated in the triple goddess, we find the first truth about Basil. She is no one simple thing...and every aspect of her is dangerous and terrifying.

Originally, the Goddess, *Oshun,* the Yoruban river goddess of West Africa, Ezulie emerged when her people were captured and taken into slavery in the Americas by white men. Since worship of pagan idols became outlawed in the Roman Catholic New Worlde, often gods and goddesses took on new faces of saints so they might still be secretly worshipped

Her parts are Ezulie Freda, Ezulie Dantor and La Siren. Often we will see her in Christian art, under different names.

Ezulie Freda

Ezulie Freda is exquisitely beautiful and is seen with white skin, blonde flowing hair and dancing green eyes. She loves the finer things in life, passion, sexual power and beauty. She is aligned with the Virgin Mary, with Aphrodite and Venus. Her favourite colour is pink and she adores sweet, lavish things, and insists that everything in her space is sparkling clean and perfumed.

Ezulie Freda knows how to turn on the feminine charm, adorning her white robes with silver. She uses her womanly wiles to her full potential. Work bores her and quite frankly, she would rather be painting her finger nails! Ezulie Freda isn't the greatest fan of women. She waves at them with her pinkie finger but, men though... she greets men folk with an amorous hug.

It is said if someone is possessed by Ezulie Freda they become flirtatious and seductive. Ezulie Freda has no time for deep involvements. She is an ardent lover, but a fickle one. She has three husbands *Damballa*, the sky father, *Ogoun*, god of war and iron, and *Agwe*, ruler of the sea. To show this she wears three wedding rings. Despite these three husbands, she is still thought to be a virgin. She loves *many* men at a time and is the Loa of gay and transgender men.

Capricious and charismatic, Ezulie Freda has enticed many lovers. Her admirers have told her many things and this she is the holder of a great many secrets. This has caused her problems though, because Ezulie Freda aims to please *every* man. So, fearing she might give up secrets when she was captured, *her own people* cut out her tongue. Now the only sounds that she can make are the ka-ka-ka-ka of the sound of her tongue clicking in the top of her mouth.

Known also as Ezulie Ge Rouge (red eyes), she cries for lost loves and things that have hurt her and is said to always leave any service held for her, crying. This is, some say, because her heart *can* never be satisfied. We can see this in her symbol the veve, a heart struck through by a dagger.

She never cries for long, though. She feels the hard side of love, the sickness hatred and rang, but she is clever. She cries out her pain rather than keeping it inside and making herself ill.

Ezulie Freda is often misunderstood as being selfish and vapid, but in truth *she* cries, so *we don't have to*. She takes on our pain. It is *her* heart pierced through by a dagger, so ours can remain whole. Perhaps one of the most misunderstood of the loa, Ezulie Freda is less called on by Voudou practitioners, because many suggest she doesn't like work and is lazy. The truth of Ezulie Freda's power though, is she expects that *you* will sort out your issues *yourself*. She is probably the most loved of all the Loa.

In the past, Haitian people would ask the Virgin Mary to call on Ezulie Freda, now in their time of emancipation, she comes to them of her own volition.

Ezulie Dantor

The second embodiment of Ezulie is the warrior goddess Ezulie Dantor. She is the **Petro** aspect of Ezulie. These are the newer, darker, aspects that rose from the goddess in the times of the Haitian slavery. Women would call out to her when their husbands beat them and slave owners overpowered and raped them.

She is driven by passion and jealousy. By contrast to Ezulie Freda, Ezulie Dantor *loves* women and will stay with them, protecting and avenging them, right through their lives. Said to have two husbands and to adore knives, she seeks terrible vengeance on those people who hurt women. The Goddess of lesbians, she is feared for her ruthlessness. Pictorially we see her depicted with deep scars on her face as testament to the battles she has fought.

Often, we might see Ezulie Dantor depicted as the Black Madonna, as she is the goddess of motherhood and, in particular, *single* motherhood. Sometimes you might see

34

her also depicted as Our Lady of Lourdes or Our Lady of Mount Carmel.

Lastly, is the erotically beautiful La Sirenne.

La Sirenne

Sea serpent and goddess of the sea, sacred and sensuous La Sirenne dances in the rivers, lakes and oceans. Her dance is the banda; lascivious and bawdy, it is beautiful, terrifying and she dances it with skill and charm. The matron saint of sailors she drinks rum laced with hot pepper sauce and screams obscenities at anyone who gets in her way. She is Maman Bridgitte a descendant of the Celtic Bridget and she is called upon to "Raise the Dead" La Sirenne is protector and guidance to anyone who is on the point of death and about to transition from this world.

My question is though, when you use basil and call on the power of Ezulie, who will arrive, Ezulie Freda, Ezulie Dantor, or the sea serpent La Sirenne?

To answer that, we need to think about the very essence of basil and how its medicine works.

The Essence of Basil

Basil is irrepressible. Inhale her from the bottle and her pervasive fragrance almost assaults the nostrils. She has no subtlety and decorum. She is a short, sharp shock. Think back to a time when you have driven back from the supermarket with a Basil plant in the car. She entirely fills the space with her scent. She borders on nauseating with how overwhelming she becomes. Everything else is drowned out by her "noise".

Botanically a *masculine* Basil plant does not exist. The plant is *gynodioecious,* that is it changes sex to always be able to reproduce alone (actually there are a very small number of male flowers amongst the female ones that make pollination possible). While Basil is female, emotionally we should say...only just! Because *Ocimum basilicum* is *not* your typical lady.

To me the moniker Sweet Basil is almost ironic. Most essential oils have gentleness, some degree of subtleness that allows healing to ethereally descend. No such luck this time. Basil doesn't care a toss about politeness.

Does it sound like I don't like her? Actually, I have come to love her but I regard her with great care – always looking out of the corner of my eye to see what she will do next; because sometimes a naughty gal is useful to have around. Let's say I treat her with a great deal of respect.

I was born during the last week of June. They call that "The Week of The Empath". What everyone around me sees as my greatest strength I regard as my harshest curse. I care too much about what other people think, say or feel. I utterly tie myself up in knots. I am sentient to a painful degree. Where my husband sees life entirely in black and white I really am... fifty shades of grey! Basil, like a focused sergeant major, mocks my cares. Screaming abuse in my ears she demands that I find the fortitude *get over myself.* As I try to bemoan the assault course my emotions are struggling with, Basil demands "Enough already. Get out of your head".

She is harsh and unfeeling. Know the saying "Got to be cruel to be kind"? Yeah, well it can often feel like she only gets the first bit! She wants you to pull yourself together because, frankly now, you are boring her. You have become tedious and she has had enough. The upside to that, of course, is you run fastest when your pants are fire...her peppery medicine certainly doesn't hang around!

In Chinese Medicine Basil is seen as drying. It is this medicine that "dries up" wet mucous in the lungs. It warms and dries creaky aching joints. Spiritually Basil says "Will you please quit being so wet!"

Sometimes a bit of pep is useful. The bullies in the playground don't run away on their own and with Basil's (sometimes uncomfortably) honest chemistry running through your veins you are made to man up and grow a pair. If you wish you flick the finger at things that are really hacking you off. Do a Basil gender switch! She doesn't care about the karma of fighting back she is just gleefully visualising the first punch. Basil believes in a taste of your own medicine...scorpion medicine!

Scorpion Medicine

Throughout the historical references we saw scorpions, serpents, sea monsters, and all manner of venomous beasts. Basil, they said, was the antidote to the venom but also caused scorpions to magically appear. I wonder why.

And yet....

The scorpion is a universal symbol that converges almost perfectly with Basil's vibrational healing.

In every ancient culture the scorpion is revered. It symbolizes transformation, strength and chaos. It speaks of self-protection and an openness to change. It signifies metamorphosis and mystery. Scorpions are independent and ferocious.

Dr Bruce Berkovsy wrote a stunning essay tying together Basil and *Androctonos,* the scorpion medicine of homeopathy. His work seems to have originated from the research done by Peter Chappell in his book *Emotional Healing with Homeopathy* where he proves the medicine of how using actual scorpion can heal certain sets of people. Andronctonus is made from the whole scorpion rather than just its venom. It is titrated and then potentised 30 times taking it to the 80th c. For those of you who are unfamiliar with homeopathy, it works on the basis of **treating like with like**. Here, this echoes the traditional African usage of frying a live scorpion and then eating it as an antidote to the progressing paralysis from a scorpion sting. Remember too, what Dioscorides told us...African people who eat Basil leaves no longer fear the pain from a scorpion's sting.

Where **aromatherapy uses extremely concentrated** essences of plants **homeopathy uses very weak** dilutions, the more diluted the treatment is taken, the more potent it becomes.

Given this *like treats like* idea then, it is interesting first to think about the scorpion itself.

Powerful and formidable warriors, scorpions were probably the first animals to leave the sea and move onto land. In over 400, 000 years, the scorpion has changed very little, making it one of the most successful evolutionary species on our planet.

They can adapt to environments in the most incredible ways, living in very harsh and extreme conditions. Able to lift up to 100 times their body weight of hard ground, they are fearsomely strong. Their resilience is unsurpassed, having incredibly efficient ways of storing water. Records show scorpions as having lived for 9 months without food or water.

Bizarrely, despite having *twelve* eyes, they also have very poor eyesight. Preferring the dark, they rarely come out in the day by choice. Their exoskeleton is a tough suit of armour and that sting in their tail can be lethal.

Scorpions prefer being alone and in the right circumstances will eat each other. Often the female will devour her mate after copulation and she will also happily feast on her children too. They have no need at all for interaction with any others of their species except for one.

Mating is an instinctual urge, a need to procreate, nothing more. The scorpion can sense the close proximity of a female by tiny delicate sensors on his legs and then will pursue her for many hours, the courtship dance being enigmatic and beautiful.

The Native Americans revere the scorpion totem as an animal of great mastery. . They admire its high self esteem, its determination and vigilance. The scorpion, they say, is intense, has strong willpower and tenacity, and that it is forceful, tranquil, and dignified.

The aboriginal culture also sees this quietness as fortitude. The scorpion's wisdom is to wait, to dig in hard and to uncover what is hidden. Its timing and calculation are essential to its survival and success. Most of all, the scorpion acts via its intuition. It senses its mate, its terrain and whether danger is near. Its medicine is in awareness and tenacity. Keep watching, keep digging, and keep working...even if nothing happens around you for many days. Patience brings results. Most of all though, to keep your instincts sharp and ready, for who knows when you might need to defend and attack.

If you do happen to find two scorpions in one place, then it is likely they are either mating, or are killing each other!

Incredibly though, scorpions seem to carry their own antidote to their venom.

In Dr Berkovsky's post he speaks of a mother who had recently stood trial in America for murdering her child, and in it he speaks of how he feels Basil resonated with the successful use of Andronctonus on sociopaths. The post reminded me of the naked courage of Lionel Shriver's *We Have to Talk about Kevin* where a child murderer's mother openly admits, whilst she loves her son, she really doesn't like him and perhaps never has. He has been far too challenging to a mother who had found breaking glass ceilings in her career effortless, and motherhood gave her challenges which she found distasteful to say the least. Loving him, now he rots in prison, takes effort and determination and she no longer feels she has the strength spare to summon.

Kevin Katchoudurian's mother, Eva, could do with a bit of Basil. You see, Basil understands cruelty and has empathy for the long fight of having lived with it. She gets it because she has being using it to manipulate people for so long.

If you have not read the book, I would urge you to do so. Not only is it exquisitely written but as novelist Max

Pearson explained "This book has given women permission to feel things that they weren't allowed to feel." Kevin at the age of 16 encompassed the very embodiment of evil, becoming a spree killer and murdering his classmates in the playground. Throughout the book it becomes clear that no matter how hard Eva searches for explanations as to why, or looks for remorse from her son, neither will be forthcoming.

This sociopathic callousness is very much the nature of Basil. And strangely just as the scorpion is believed to carry an antidote to its *own* venom, Basil seems to be an antidote for *these people* too. It is a medicine against their *own qualities* but also against the *emotional wreckage* they leave behind. Actually, the terms **psychopath** and **sociopath** are more blanket pop culture terms and these people should more correctly fall under heading **Antisocial Personality Disorder**. Whilst it might be comforting to imagine these are people we are unlikely to come into contact with, in everyday life, the statistics sadly state otherwise. It is thought that psychopaths make up about 1% of general population and 4% have sociopathic tendencies. (That said, it is notoriously difficult to study these people because they so enjoy manipulating and skewing tests!)

Sociopaths are defined as having some combination of the following:

- Failure to conform to social norms

- Deceptiveness

- Impulsivity

- Irritability

- Reckless irresponsibility

- Lack of remorse

Where psychopaths are *born*, sociopaths are thought to be *made*. The result of their childhood environment, they may have suffered at the hands of harsh and inconsistent parenting. Often parents might have been involved in substance abuse whether that is drink or drugs, research also shows that often their mothers had smoked when they were pregnant too.

If there is someone in your life whom you suspect might fall under this banner, look to the very beginning of your relationship for the clues. They will have lied; lied about their job, their family and their social standing. Over time the lies will become more and more outrageous and eventually, in hindsight you might start to wonder how you fell for them. But boy is he plausible and his charm will draw you in. You might also be alerted to how few people are around him. Sociopaths aren't able to maintain emotional ties, not least because they are incapable of feeling shame, guilt or remorse about some of the horrible things they have done to people!

Actually, he doesn't give a monkey's fig about other people's feelings, because he is used to getting his own way and this is always his ultimate end game. To do this, he will use charm and charisma and he will always be found basking in the spotlight, holding court, centre stage.

Often you might hear a partner speak of her ex as being a sociopath or a narcissist, and, again we are in the Basil garden here. The two are closely aligned but have different motivations behind them. Narcissistic Personality Disorder affects around 6.2% of the population with a higher prevalence in men. Incidentally, I will state here that whilst I said "he" with sociopaths, that might just as likely be a she. For balance, we'll have a she to demonstrate the narcissists, not least because there has been a great deal of research done into the daughters of narcissistic mothers and how it affects their subsequent lives.

The narcissist doesn't really feel the need to lie because she is more than happy with her mental attributes and appearance. Her vanity is enough for her to expect that you *should* put her on a pedestal. Selfish and vain, these people genuinely expect that the world should revolve around them – their sole motivation in life is to garner praise and approval from everyone they meet. The slightest criticism and they will cut you to the core. Your feelings don't come into it. It is all about how they feel and what you did *to them*. Oft, these are very intellectually gifted people and they feel that they should be at the top of their career. God forbid you are the person that gets in their way because a stiletto on the career ladder really will hurt...and if that's what she thinks it will take... then prepare yourself for the pain.

Many people misunderstand the motivation of the narcissist as someone who s simply absorbed by their looks but there is a far deeper complexity to the disorder and most certainly it is a spectrum. There are those who have mild dimensions of it to their personality (if not all of us, in fact!) and there are those who are very severely afflicted. And to me it does feel like an affliction because it is a dark dis-ease. Narcissists can plummet into extremely black holes of despair. Often they suffer terrible self esteem issues. Not least, because many are the children of narcissists themselves. They have grown up with totally unreal expectations put on their head. Their childhoods were probably pendulums swings between vast praise and totally being ignored, because they were not reflecting their parent's glory at the time.

The narcissist becomes a master manipulator to survive. Their carefully crafted skill is "look at me". Healthily you might see them on a stage, or rocking a football stadium to a beat...unhealthily is a nasty history of cruelty and bad behaviour and a whole host of loved ones in tears by the way side.

Recognition is her sole objective and the second you remove your attention from her validation, expect her to start plotting your comeuppance. She is vengeful and vindictive. She will be looking to channel her venom. Actually it might not always be apparent but this need for recognition is to stroke *her* endless cry for reassurance. When finally you think "Enough is enough" you will find they begin to chase. They get nastier, boundaries are smashed and your personal space will be gone.

Much like our scorpion there is always the danger of unprovoked attack.

Funnily enough a post on *thenarcissistschild.com* regales Aesop's fable as a demonstration what it is like to live with one of these people. A scorpion and a frog meet on the bank of a stream and the scorpion asks the frog to carry him across on its back. The frog asks, "How do I know you won't sting me?" The scorpion says, "Because if I do, I will die too."

The frog is satisfied, and they set out, but in midstream, the scorpion stings the frog. The frog feels the onset of paralysis and starts to sink, knowing they will both drown, but he has just enough time to gasp "Why?"

"Because," replies the scorpion: "It is my nature..."

And I can't think of a truer depiction, but it also demonstrates why Basil is such a powerful friend to family members of these people. Whilst the "normal" amongst us are desperately trying to the follow the thread that shows us what on earth we did to deserve this, Basil tells you "Well, it's just because..."

Enough already....get out of your head.

Do you remember the scene from Sex in the City where Miranda has a complete epiphany when two girls explain "He just isn't into you"? She was entirely liberated by the simplicity of it. She hadn't done anything wrong, the analysis could stop, and for a narcissist's child Basil's medicine feels the same.

Physically Basil is cephalic, it clears the brain. Mentally though, it feels like someone opened all the windows in your head and let the rubbish fly out. Lawless describes Basil as being second only to rosemary; to a certain extent I agree. If you want to focus your mind, concentrate, or even make decisions more clearly then rosemary *is* top dog. But if you just want the emotional merry go round to stop, if you want to quit with the "*what-ifs*", or if you want to have an "*I'll show you*" moment, where just for a second, you don't consider the consequences, then trust Basil will turn up wearing khakis and combats and I promise you she will have your back. Say it loud, say it proud and then walk away. Hopefully your scorpion will do what nature demands of it, and he will disappear back under his rock!

It is potent medicine because just once in a while it is very healthy to say your piece.

But, just as the scorpion's sting is conditioned, so the narcissist's child begins a similar pattern. Always mindful that they are playing with an erstwhile unexploded bomb they develop their own stinging mechanism too. For months, they unwittingly run scripts in their heads ready for the pin to be pulled. Aware that no matter how nice their loved one can be, there will always be a payback, very soon they become vicious too. So again Basil is helpful here.

When I have read more into Andronctonus, other uses have resonated with me about Basil too. Some discuss the poor parents who are terrified of their ADD child. They wrangle with ways to try to parent the child who feels entirely alone in the world and fights tooth and nail to keep it that way. How did the child they had so gently held in their arms become so entirely devoid of trust and empathy with anyone? How did he become so detached from the norm? I am sure this a question so many people desperately plead as they cry themselves to sleep.

I found two pieces of information that made think more deeply about this. In my mum's book *The Garden of Eden* (Jill Bruce) says of Basil:

There is an affinity with the spinal cord and it seems to remove emotional blocks around the cord and especially the neck. It removes the blocks and lifts up the brain.

Dr. Jean Valnet quotes the work of Cadéac and Meunier as proof that Basil first stimulates then lessens cerebro activity. I can feel the pent up anger of so many years of manipulation travelling down my spine and making me a want to lash out...but somewhere between the brain and my stinging tail the need to strike seems to dissipate with Basil. (Child or arachnid...who can tell?!)

Usually, I place the prayer of gratitude at the end of the book, but in this book the vibrational healing of Basil is exactly this:

God, grant me the serenity
to accept the things I cannot change,
the courage to change the things I can,
and the wisdom to know the difference.

Reinhold Niebuhr

Acceptance does not have to mean being the victim. For many people the only antidote to living with these people is to finally excise them from their lives. But life is complex and sometimes that might be impossible. Whilst you are waiting for the universe to catch up, let Basil mark your boundaries.

In his book, *The Earthwise Herbal: A Complete Guide to Old World Medicinal Plants*, Matthew Wood cites the work of Brent Davis using Basil to treat patients who had been using marijuana. Davis had noted that this was traditional usage of the plant both in India and in the Middle East. Over time he noticed that the typical patient would become increasingly convinced that their body was deteriorating and feared their health was permanently compromised. Interestingly he describes how, regardless of spinal manipulation, there seemed to be a weakness in the ligaments that never seemed to correct itself and he came to believe that the problem might be due to some sort of "nervous disorganisation" Not only did he recommend Basil for the removal of herbal medicines lodged in the tissues but chemical ones too.

Potentially I might be over stating a point here, but just in case it has been missed...what do we know about a large number of parents of sociopaths? Could the residue of the wretched childhoods they gave to their children, smoking a joint, be erased simply by a herb? I would think not...but I'd still be shoving pesto on my partner's pasta at every given opportunity if it were me!

One last point here, you just ask Jeremy Kyle what marijuana does to the mind. *Paranoid?* Basil issues its favourite ultimatum... *Get Out of Your Head!*

One anomaly struck me in the homeopathic proving of adronctonus; the repeated discussion of how noise seemed to aggravate the patient. They found it overly irritating. This seems to be spookily close to the medieval usage that one should use Basil in a child's ear for earache. It also made me think of the overwhelming need to go away and hide from noise when you have a migraine (which basil is excellent for) ...oh and to find a dark place to go and hade from the world too.

Lastly, I think it is worth noting the statement "psychopaths are born, but sociopaths are made". I don't think it is too dangerous to say we all have these tendencies to a greater and lesser degree. Life events can make us nicer or not such nice people. And whilst I am not saying we all turn into sociopaths when life gets hard...we can take on some of their tendencies, the lying, the cheating and playing two ends against the middle. With or without the psychiatric label, the actions still hurt. Better have a bottle of Basil at the ready.

Mars Medicine

Astrologically Basil is ruled by the planet Mars and also by his Grecian counterpart Aries. And just like all the confusing misdirection we have with the sociopath/narcissist issues; we have a weird contradiction here too. Mars is the Roman god of conquest, the son of Jupiter. He was revered by the Romans above all others. Aries however, does not have anywhere as nice a connotation about him as Mars. He is seen to be irrational, unpredictable and *warmongering*. (It kind of reminds me of "You started that, now I'm going to finish it..." We have the feeling that someone steps in and decides *enough already!*)

Mars is the planet through which the divine self expresses itself. It is the ego. This is because it is the planet closest to spirit. Think of Aries, the baby of the newly born zodiac year. The infant sign in vital and yet untainted by life's experience.

Mars is assertive, purposeful and self expressive. It is very pure energy uninfluenced by thought or emotion...it just is like a hurricane rushing through your life. It is a vitally important planet because whilst the rest of the solar system is sitting around contemplating their navels, Mars says come on. Let's see you do it then. There is no "inner work" with Mars. He is all about the physical, about action. There will always be an expectation that you *do* something about a situation.

We would all love to drift on a millpond of calm but Mars's unsettling energy is welcome because he ushers survival instinct, work and sheer impetus to move forward. He is ambition, achievement and, of course, he is conquest.

You'll never find Mars inside of the mental fortress. He's not a thinker. You'll find him outside of the spirit realm defending the king or queen. What's more he is spirit's right hand man; it is he who does the bidding. In the same way your sensibilities, hopes and dreams dwell inside of that castle. If anyone starts to mess with your head, Mars says "clear off, I'm in charge here." He'll protect them. If he feels you are not paying heed to what's wanted inside of "the castle" best look out...because he *will* wage war on you. His loyalty will be offended by anyone's audacity to question, and you'll feel his fiery energy come into play. Arguments, fights, sheer bloody mindedness...these are signs Mars has decided to step in.

He's not an antagonist though. Not a rebel, anarchist or even Machiavellian. He doesn't *need* to stir up trouble to prove his worth. He knows *instinctively* that he is important. (Aye aye! Another narcissist, just what we need!) His warrior spirit **only kicks in through defence**.

Spirit yearns for you to express yourself with integrity. She wants you to instinctively feel what is right for you and speak your truth, being authentic to that. Keep your counsel for too long though, and I assure you she will have something to say. She will get sick of being oppressed, whisper to conspiratorially Mars about it (and you know what Mars feels about oppressors.) But, make no mistake, when finally you start to speak your truth she will dance in tribute to your cause.

And it is useful, I think, to remember that Basil resonates on the throat chakra, that energy centre governing communication and expression. Think about the effects of a closed down throat chakra; we might see the repetitive irritating cough of the woman who suspects her sister might be abused – but was frightened to say anything. Or another who feels very disappointed by her lot, but would never tell her husband so. Silently she washes up and yet strangely feels the need to keep clearing her throat. Does the quick anti-tussive (stops coughing) action of Basil becomes Mars demanding:

"Spit it out woman!"?

Often we see these emotions swallowed up because we don't want to hurt another, but over time the petty angst becomes very real anguish indeed.

So here is where the difficulties start, because is Mars anger? Is he rage? Well no. He can't be, can he? Because he is simply...energy.

So these more difficult emotions start to rear their heads when Mars energy has been repressed. After a while we get annoyed, then we get angry and if it is the right time of the month we get goddamn furious!!!

Mars in balance is brute force. Mars *out* of balance is temper tantrums. What's exciting is that energy is not only destructive but it can be also virulently creative. It brings about change. It is fertile, orgasmic and powerful. Mars is like the toddler that wants to build, build, build, and because his ambition is so fierce he wants his tower to be taller than anyone ever built it before. He will be the conqueror.

Funnily enough, astrologically, the first time Mars re-visits the point it was at in a natal chart when a child was born, is at 26 months old. The terrible twos! Mars magic in all its most beautifully uncomfortable majesty! Baby is into everything. He has found his feet and he wants to explore.

He's smashing every toy he's got. There are bells, tambourines, drums, smash, smash, smash. He wants to taste and experience everything!

And he develops his very favourite word.

Nnnno!

He is learning to separate himself from his parents. This is the first time he has experienced independence and he loves it. Goddess forbid anyone gets in his way....Mars energy, Basil energy.

But sometimes of course, Mars can be a bit too much. You ask any mother whose child has made to 27 months! She'll look at you tired and bedraggled and smile wanly at everyone who has the audacity to say "Oh isn't he adorable!"

Mars out of balance might not only be the patient who is afraid to speak her truth, but it can also be like the toddler who hasn't grasped the naughty step yet. He's a bit too forceful, a bit too in your face, because imbalance is imbalance *whichever way the pendulum swings....*

If there is to be a personification of Basil working in balance, she is a peacekeeper in Afghanistan. In the heat, she is fearless, brave and discriminating. She fights for the rights of the underdog. She is loyal and completely reliable. She has trained until her skills are faultless. Months of being drilled means she can make decisions in the blink of an eye. She doesn't have time for moral discourse. Kill or be killed (Oil, soldier, scorpion.)

Ezulie Dantor...

You see it is very easy for us to make moral judgements and ethical arguments when we sit at home in front of the TV. She is out there living it. And thank God for her, because our lives are made so much richer for her. She is not gentle, she is tough and my goodness we need her. But remember; don't mistake her attack strategy as aggressive. She never is. Always defensive...at checkpoints with a gun, lurking by rocks with a stinging tail, arguing from a narcissistic point of view....Basil medicine is always from defence. It's quick, sharp and decisive. And if you deserve it...GOOD!

Often, I see Basil described as an uplifting oil, but again this feels a bit too floaty for this stroppy herb. She is more like the friend who tells you to get your glad rags on, takes you by the hand and drags you out on the town. She is a bit shameless and utterly delicious for it. She'll encourage you to do all manner of things that you'll regret in the morning but boy it feels fab at the time. There will be fun though. Look out on the dance floor. Basil'll be rocking it out - beer bottle held high, demonstrating every syllable of

Sisters are doing it for themselves.... You can see it reverberating right to her very core.

I have become very interested in how essential oils help the mind. In particular how we might be able to use them as a medicine to emancipate the spirit. As an example let's have a show of hands. How many of you have husbands who worry themselves stupid about being at work in the school holidays. Do *they* feel guilty about leaving their kids? I can't imagine there would be many hands go up to that question. But what about if I ask how many other women feel that way? I suspect it will be more.

That's not a judgement on men. Rather a comment on our emotional biology. Perhaps we, as women, have not yet evolved defences to help us in these societal roles. Maybe we are not supposed to. Either way, hormones get in the way. So we have all these choices that were kept from us until a hundred years ago. To work, to vote, to defend our country, to parent in different ways... but do we really have choices at all? Most of the time the mortgage company is *our* dictator...but we also suffer pressure from those around us too.

So we do what we think we should, but most of the time it doesn't make us happy, but the bills have been paid.

But what if....we just said "f**k it"

(Incidentally I have just been breathing the oil for some weeks now and it is taking every ounce of myself discipline not to take those asterisks out. There's a naughtiness building in side!)

What about if we listened to the impish spirit, with her arms folded scowling and stamping her feet "I don't *want* to" and heeded what she had to say.

That would be bad.

Or would it?

Well, that's the million dollar question isn't it?

Basil requires that I state her case, and who am I to argue. (Not bloody likely!)

Many cultures give the same magickal attribution to Basil, that you should put a sprig in the cash register to attract prosperity. So let's for a second imagine that we did that. We picked a sprig, put it in the drawer and closed up for the night. As we sleep she releases her oil. The linalool builds. The vapours are trapped.

Next morning, open the drawer and the medicine explodes into the atmosphere.

Her drive. Her determination. Her devil may care attitude. Her astute decision, passion, focus, black and white discrimination, practiced precision, expertise, creativity, ingenuity, protection, loyalty...

Act. Act. Act.

Get out of your head woman. *Just do it!!!*

Now just for a second, let's gently close the drawer. Can you hear the kindly souls we are usually surrounded by, whispering: "Don't push yourself too hard" "We just don't want you to get your hopes up" "It's harder for women...?"

Blimey! Someone make a sale so I can cop a whiff of Basil again.

Hmmmm, I think I might be starting to see her point.

You see, if you have a glass ceiling in your head that it stopping you from achieving, then Basil's your gal. All those prejudices you have carried about working women, all your self-doubt, all the emotional clutter of spelling bees, shopping lists, making dinner, well they fly out the window. All that is left is pure Mars energy. Pure spiritual drive. Pure essence...and it goes off like a search missile. Better move out of the way because glass smithereens are going to be pouring around you for weeks. You'll wonder what the hell just happened. Those around you will watch open mouthed.

Basil will defend your right to be who or what you want to be. Your right to make a living, if that's what you want to do. Your right to do exactly what makes your spirit soar....remember, her mars energy means she is closer to it than any other oil. Basil is very much a grown up with a temper tantrum never far away....

Standing on her own two feet

Ringing on her own bells

And I like that. It frightens the pants off me. But I like it.

So, the question in mind now must be...what catalyst exists within Basil to neutralise this venom. Where is this alchemy coming from?

The Basil touchstone is through its rulership by Scorpio, the sign of transformation.

Scorpio Medicine

Basil is also ruled by the astrological constellation of Scorpio. Strangely Scorpio is also ruled by Mars and again we have this strange contradiction that, whilst Mars is most definitely masculine, Scorpio is a feminine sign. Here, like the Mars/ Aries collaboration we have another sign that gets bad press. If I say to someone I am a Cancerian you can almost feel them want to pat me on the head, because we are cute, cuddly and mumsy and then, of course, there is also the cake!

But Scorpio...?

Not so much.

Immediately people think of that sting in the tail. It is all a bit unfair really because there is so much more to Scorpio (and I have to be nice because my mother in law is Scorpio...and for the record I think she is one of the loveliest people that ever walked the planet, so I'll fight Scorpio's corner!)

Astrologically Scorpio represents a pivotal place in life's path. That juxtaposition between life and death, and it has intimate associations with both. In England, as we welcome the Scorpio birthdays at the end of October, night and day are fairly evenly balanced, but every day we walk through the sign, darkness encroaches more. The plants and animals retreat for the winter, the crisp leaves fall, and the trees become bare. We enter a time of quietness and regeneration. The leaves fall, but their rotting and decomposition will only serve to feed the tree. It absorbs the goodness of the death. Darkly, Scorpio has strong associations with the underworld, most specifically with the unconscious and with one's instinctive nature. Because of this Scorpio, and by extension its daughter plant Basil, provide a very fertile land for transformation.

The keynote terms for anything that falls under Scorpio rule are *test, trial and triumph*. Most certainly we see Scorpio channelling her medicine through Basil in an enigmatic and powerful way. It transforms ones desires by conquering fears and doubts. And suddenly we can see how Mars medicine can come to the fore, because Scorpio changes the internal narratives.

For the most part, a Scorpio ruled plant is not for everyday use. Consider it to be like a burglar alarm, mace spay or fire extinguisher. We use them in times of crises. Think *test, trial,* triumph because the key to triumph is always going to be re-orientation. In the darkness, all of our usual resources are taken and suddenly we have to live on our wits. Only here can our instinctual nature overtake our conscious mind.

Can you think of a time when life was unbelievably hard and you felt there were no options left? In order to "get out of jail free" you needed to rethink, consider possibilities you might not have thought of, create something out of nothing? That is most definitely Scorpio medicine.

Scorpio is also viewed as the success planet and looking at it from this new fresher perspective, this Scorpio Basil medicine is where we find these amazing sparks of creativity. Here, in these dark times is where our instincts kick in and where our unconscious smiles and says...Aaah! You remember what I am for now, do you?

Because when life is easy, we become complacent. We do what serves us well and we sail that happy millpond. But when life challenges us, then we step up a gear. This inherent survival instinct kicks in and the warrior emerges. And then, only then, we truly see what we are made of. The scorpion sheds its outgrown exoskeleton and something newer, more powerful and resourceful steps out.

So, raising the Scorpio pennant high into the air, what is the positive message of the sign? Follow it for dramatic intensity and focused direction of your purpose. March to the beat of its drum to start to see a far greater significance to your life and suddenly find real endurance skills and enormous stamina to complete your task...whatever it takes. With the Basil/ Scorpio leadership there is a hungry chase for the goal which stays permanently in your sights. You feel ultimately determined and the pursuit of your goal is truly relentless. Scorpio is self contained and very concentrated. It is very rare you are unable to achieve what you set out to accomplish when you have Scorpio/Basil on your side.

But when the sun rises high in the sky, a charred hotness of Scorpio medicine is caught in the shade of its flag. When Basil is used too regularly or in overly high dilutions one might consider its effects to be a little like Mickey Mouse in The Sorcerer's Apprentice. He wields his magic with excitement and gusto, but it far exceeds his capabilities. This is very much the tone of Scorpio medicine gone mad, it literally takes control of you. Scorpio passion is dark, controlling and secretive.

Here we will find stubbornness, of course, but jealousy too. Often Scorpio can be uncommunicative. Always cunning, it is possessive, suspicious and manipulative. It is not unusual to see a strong and brutal sexual nature. There is violence, sarcasm, vindictive emotions and cynical and devious measures.

Interestingly, Scorpio is often described as the actor of the zodiac because it is seen as an artist able to play on the emotions of others. Imagine him to be an actor in a drama. The audience is caught up in his melodrama and will laugh and cry with him. At the end of the play they leave feeling elated because the play has been cathartic for them. They have experienced joy and pain but, thank Goddess, not their own.

This is very much a Scorpio thing and again we shall say Basil thing too; this idea of emotions whose magnitude are so enormous they cannot be put into words. So, instead of having to find a voice for them and thus needing to experience them, often there are words, easier to find, that will cause *other* people to feel your pain instead. Rudeness, spite, warmongering...

Scorpio quakes at the idea of bringing these wretched feelings to the surface and so, often, the distraction of an outburst serves the occasion far more comfortably. Scorpio understands how devastating it can be to actually *own* those feelings, terrified you might be consumed by their flames....better to enact rather than fall victim to their pain. So when the words literally get stuck in your throat and you start acting out...kicking other kids, bullying, or even just avoiding a pertinent subject, Scorpio closes the throat. Use Basil to open it.

What's interesting to me is that being dramatic is cathartic for some people, and for others it is simply pretence, and so I wonder why this is? What is the thrill of all this secrecy and pretence? Perhaps living multiple lives means not having to face a world that is either too mundane or too painful for them to bear.

Scorpio medicine forces us to face our limitations in order that we can evolve past them. Plants that come under Scorpio rule (myrrh, Melissa, garlic, nettle, thistle, mustard, wild lettuce and thuja) ask us to make choices about what we want to do with past patterns inhabiting our psyche. They open doors and say "Are you ready to leave this one behind, or are you more comfortable with the status quo as it is?".

Clearly these are not easy choices. Even the most toxic situations can feel terrifying to leave behind, but Basil and its partners line up like an army of support here, quietly pushing back the riot of thoughts clamouring to break forth, keeping them in line so you could pass through, if you so desired. Most importantly remember Scorpio is a very fertile sign, not in the idea of making babies, but in the concept of personal growth. Consider her to be tilling the soil to get rid of these patterns of stagnation and non-growth to bring about a catalyst of change that will move you forward.

Scorpio is also the planet of the subject of psychology in its complete entirety. It is the sign that brings about the most self knowledge, not least because it *insists* we plunge to the depths to find out exactly what lies beneath: dreams, the things we don't own up to thinking, our jealousies and insecurities, but most pertinently the parts of us that we absolutely loathe. It is important medicine because how can we know what we are made of unless we understand our shadow side as well as those parts we don't mind other people seeing? Basil wants to know what makes us tick and why.

As such Basil medicine also demands that you ask yourself "*why?*"

"Why is that winding me up so much?"

"What happened there that I got so upset?" "Where exactly is that button wired back to, that causes me to act like this?"

Without a shadow of doubt, these are not going to be good places but Basil seems to be able to anaesthetise them, and in my experience seems to be able to make the explanation so simple that when the words come out of your mouth you go...was that it? And it's gone.

To the uninitiated it might feel frightening to enter the world of Basil, and I would say *astute observation*, because unless you understand the plant, be sure that it will become your master. Basil and Scorpio are always on the lookout for hidden motives and agendas; not least because when Scorpio energy has been repressed for a long time it can unconsciously project onto other people around you (remember how the actor works?). Certainly there will always be this element of paranoia.

To consider using Basil it is useful to bring to mind the words of Sun Tzu from *The Art of War*.

"If you know the enemy and know yourself, you need not fear the result of a hundred battles. If you know yourself but not the enemy, for every victory gained you will also suffer a defeat. If

you know neither the enemy nor yourself, you will succumb in every battle."

Basil medicine, Scorpio medicine and particularly that of Ezulie Freya expects that *you* will turn up to do the work. *You* will understand that <u>you hold the answers.</u> It is you that will have to change ***<u>because ultimately you are the only person you have control over.</u>***

It is a good job we have Mars medicine here too, because it takes real courage to face these demons; to lift the rock and find out how many other scorpions are lying beneath. Illuminating these painful moments brings real liberation of the spirit, but when you do, then just think of the magic that small bottle wields. Suddenly, with the doors to new solutions open, the light floods in and you can no longer run and hide in the shadows. Then you have to learn a new strategy, and so with Basil's help... you do.

Self reliance, patience, emotional stability, calmness and objectivity all become new weapons in the arsenal to replace that sting in your tail. Most of all, you absorb the very un-Scorpio skill of waiting to see how things will pan out without resorting to the usual emotional outbursts that will normally manifest.

I like to think of it as "coming out the other side" of these times. It helps me to imagine they will always end and there is light at the end of the tunnel. At the end of a Scorpio lesson, you will always have learned a lot; about you, and about the motivations of others around you. The gift of Scorpio medicine is that from it you can become an incredible healer of some description. You have knowledge of the human condition that helps you to support others you may meet. You have unravelled the mysteries and most importantly, you lived to fight another day.

Most commonly, when a planet has a Scorpio dimension to it, there will be a theme where the healing encourages you **to try to get to the bottom of things**, to dig up the root cause (And don't forget how much soil our arachnid friend can lift, so it is *predictable* that Basil will expect you to do an inordinate amount of work.)

Scorpio says "We can do this the easy way or the hard way...but we are going to do this" It will insist that you stop hiding from things, stop searching and just face the feelings you have been trying to avoid, and like the Rabbi brings the truth of God, this final judgement of your own perceived failings feels like a self exorcism, and that can't be bad.

So when we plunge to these Scorpio depths what can we expect to find? Well, the terrifying truth is we *know* what lies there. It is that black cauldron of self hatred that all of us have, to some greater or lesser degree. Those doors we keep firmly shut in our heads, for fear of releasing a poisonous tidal wave of our perceived failings. We dread exposing a rush of insights, so hideous, they are capable of harming us forever. We live in fear that we might never recover from its acidic embrace. For many of us there is a very real concern that they might kill us completely and so it becomes sensible to lock that door shut, double lock it and move as far away as we can from it.

And yet....

Many of the studies into self hatred exist because there is a need to better understand substance abuse and addiction. Common themes raising their heads on the pathway to recovery are often self judgement, self attack, incredibly low self esteem and hideous self loathing.

One of the influential factors in addiction is avoidance. Addicts learn coping strategies to enable them to skirt around issues, suppress feelings and even negate them entirely. They become experts at hiding from their true self because they cannot face who they perceive that they are.

They become convinced that any feelings of upset, disappointment or rage must be wrong, inaccurate, unwanted or even inappropriate and they take steps to do whatever it takes not to feel them.

Pop psychology tells us that self compassion is the answer to our prayers; the route out of our personal hell. A recent paper published in *Psychoneuroendocrinology Journal* backed up this claim proving self compassion reduces cortisone levels and ten in turn promotes oxytocin which is known to reduce cravings in the context of substance abuse, but in our context it also brings about a happier glow and aids social interaction.

I was surprised to find that self loathing actually has a clinical name. They call it *autophobia* and it is a treatable condition. But where the Facebook posts lose credibility is they infer that the antidote to self loathing is self love. That if we say that we are fantastic enough times then we will believe it to be true and thus it is. The truth is that, self love is the <u>result</u> of the therapy and work put in, not the *route* to it.

<u>Crying</u> is the missing mechanism. Facing the pain, letting it engulf you, experiencing and letting it pass on.

You ask Ezulie Freya, and she'll bring you some tears! Grieving for and accepting the part these hurts have had in your life, and acknowledging they are not your fault. Finding a way to realise that even though you might have times in your life when you have failed, **_you_** are not a failure...and I have to say Basil does that.

It makes you look at your life in a very critical way, but there is the essence of "Is it was it is. Perhaps now it is time to move on"

An interesting theory I read about healing self loathing was to challenge the patterns that we make. We have seen this through the book haven't we? Acting out. Hurting other people so that we don't have to feel it ourselves. The theory being that the purpose of the pattern is to stop the need for the avoided feelings from resurfacing. So what can we do to break the cycle then?

Well, the suggestions are to try to be aware of signals when you are about to head off into one of your patterns and do something physical to interrupt the pattern. Jump up and dance, do some painting or put on a piece of music that you know will make you cry. I would say sniff some Basil oil. The idea is not to distract the mind, but rather to stop it in its tracks so the "auto" gets challenged to realign.

Other suggestions are to argue your case against the internal conversations, so when we hear "I'm useless" whispering through our mind, we physically open our mouths and explain all the reasons why that doesn't make sense.

Another psychology journal suggested that many of us give far too much credibility to what goes on in our heads. We listen to that voice that says we are not good enough and believe it must be true, because common sense suggests we know ourselves better than everyone else. The chances are, though, that we simply don't see the same reflections of ourselves everyone else sees, and perhaps it is time to start trusting that other people's more generous opinions of us might be happier and healthier ones to accept. Since negative and positive attributes can coalesce, and our personalities don't have straight lines of context, why not simply absorb their ideals of us, rather than use those we don't like about ourselves to define ourselves.

A particular strategy I found amusing and thus would probably work really well for me is to agree with the voice and then outtalk it making the dire consequences of how useless I am get bigger and bigger until even my own mind laughs at how ridiculous it is being. I think I already like the person who came up with this!

However you tackle the cauldron, when Basil reveals it, is up to you. But if you embrace Scorpios challenge then this self hatred will shake loose and leave. And that leaves space for love. Self love and love of every other kind available to you. Close your eyes and breathe it in. Fill the dark void that has been left and fill it with light.

Basil as an Aphrodisiac

For generations, right across the globe Basil has been connected to love. Often you will also see her listed as an aphrodisiac too. Probably to mention that Mars / phallus connection is obvious but I think it has a bearing here.

Basil medicine is so hot and spicy sometimes it canalmost feel like the energy of a one night stand, but in the context of a marriage where the sex life has become a bit screwed-up this is very healthy medicine. There is none of the play acting, manipulation, and power games that sexual issues invite. It encourages a clear and honest "I want to make love to you" and that's it. Funny how those words are so simple and yet often many of us will design elaborate seductions and facades surrounding them. Simple, straight forward, yang energy taking-the-initiative Basil. *Get out of your head.*

Most usually you will see Basil listed as a method of securing faithfulness from a loved one. None of that seems to sit very well with our scorpion gal though does it?

But if the old tenet "keep him interested" rings true, then maybe it does. Remember Mars alone has none of the romance of roses. More the seduction of a courtesan. Of Lola Montez perhaps?

While I have been writing this book the Volbeat song about the courtesan has rung out everywhere and I while I have been head banging along loving it I hadn't heard a word except for "wherever she walks". Didn't even know the name of the song...!

But there she was my scorpion girl singing at me from every speaker. I had never even heard of the "Shady and tempered dame". A real person! You could have knocked me over with a feather.

The Irish Spanish dancer (originally born Maria Dolores Eliza Rosanna Gilbert) came to pull the strings of the German government and throne. She captivated the world with her beauty, her fierce personality and an erotic spider dance. But it was not her dancing that ever made her famous but her temper and bad behaviour.

Born into a well connected Irish family in 1821 "Eliza's" family quickly moved to Liverpool and then to India. Having lost her husband very young when he died of cholera, her mother remarried another officer who cared for Eliza very well, but he was bothered by her often wild behaviour and so she was moved from school to school. At 16, the young Eliza eloped, but her marriage, in Calcutta only lasted for five years. Eliza took to the stage as a dancer under the pseudonym Lola Montez. Sadly she was recognised as the wife of Lieutenant James and the scandal drove her out of India onto the continent. She re-assumed her dancing, but her great beauty and dreadful temper far outshone her talents. But her wild charisma entranced the gentlemen and soon, Lola Montez was a well sought after courtesan.

She had originally tried to re-launch her career in the dance houses in Paris, and had caught the eye of the composer Franz Liszt. He had introduced Lola into the bohemian social circles of George Sand, French novelist and amoré of Frederick Henry Chopin. Lola enchanted the intelligentsia in the Paris salons. When in 1845, her lover newspaper editor Alexandre Dujarier was killed in a duel (not over her, it seems!) Lola left Paris and headed to Germany. To Munich.

Here she was to enchant King Ludwig I of Bavaria. Legend has it than when he asked her, in public, if her bosom was real she tore open her bodice to prove, to everyone present, that it was. Beguiled by the woman, Ludwig soon made her countess of Bavaria and granted her annuity. And bit by bit "that Montez woman" began to wield more and more political power, all of the time offending people everywhere, with her arrogant and rude manner. Lobbying for liberalism against the conservatives and the Jesuits, she became a political powerhouse and was successful in bringing down the entire administration of the Karl von Abel, one of the most powerful statesmen of the time.

Students at the university were outraged at the influence Lola was exerting and rumours began to speak of an uprising. At Lola's advice the king closed the university. When 1848 it did eventually reopen, Ludwig had a revolution on his hands. He abdicated and she fled Bavaria.

Having had many relationships and adventures in Switzerland and America, Lola headed for Australia.

Hired to the Theatre Royal, Melbourne in September1855 she performed a dance that was to make her name in history. Much to the horror of the audience she was reputed to have raised her skirt so high, in her spider dance, that everyone could see she was utterly devoid of underwear (In fact, historical evidence shows these were salacious rumours, easy to spread given her reputation). But when respectable families started to boycott the theatre, the venue's days were numbered.

In another show, she delighted 400 gold miners to a standing ovation with her charismatic performance only to subsequently offend them by then bombarding them with insults by return! Her notoriety only grew more, when performing in Ballarat, she read a rather unpleasant review about her show. So, in response she attacked the editor Henry Seekamp with a whip, and if that isn't scorpion medicine I don't know what is!!!

By 1856 Lola had had her fill of Australia and headed to San Francisco where we start to see her calm down. In 1859, The Philedelphia press reported that she was:

living very quietly up town, and doesn't have much to do with the world's people. Some of her old friends, the Bohemians, now and then drop in to have a little chat with her, and though she talks beautifully of her present feelings and way of life, she generally, by way of parenthesis, takes out her little tobacco pouch and makes a cigarette or two for self and friend, and then falls back upon old times with decided gusto and effect. But she doesn't tell anybody what she's going to do"

She remained unpredictable then right up until her death in 1861. Even at her very end her scorpion ways seemed to hold true when on 30th June 1860 she suffered a stroke and then suffered partial paralysis (even that feels like a string from the tail!) Recovering enough to be able to go outside for a stroll, finally our tragic but captivating heroine contracted pneumonia (it was always going to be her lungs wasn't it – poor soul) and after a month of fighting died.

Wherever she walks

She'll be captivating all the men

Don't look in her eyes

You might fall and find the love of your life heavenly

But she'll catch you in her web

The love of your life, yeah.

Feel the fire where she walks...oh yes that's Basil all right.

The songwriter concludes with

Oh Lola I'm sure that the love would have been

The key to all your pain

The key to all your pain

No words will later come

Did the spider bite your tongue

We will surely not forget

We will surely not forget

The Lola spider dance

The poor narcissist and her fight for the love she so fiercely feels she deserves. Eventually poison overtakes her.

Yes I know someone like that. Do you?

Actually I have known a few and every one of them has damaged me to some small degree. And what's saddest is they are the ones who stay with us. The ones who write the scripts we ruin our lives by. They do catch us in their webs of deceit until we are entirely trapped. The songwriter's right. They're ones we never really forget.

And so are we faithful...?

We stay ever entwined if that's the same thing.

If it is... then I don't think I want it. Do you?

Now, let's just for a second think about the mind body spirit dynamic of how Basil works on the respiratory system. Well first of all, we need to acknowledge the speed of her healing. Literally, she cuts through mucous like a knife. But what caused it to be there in the first place? Infection clearly, but why did the weakness happen in the lungs? Might it be a throat chakra mechanism from swallowing ones emotions? Or perhaps there is so much talking, but none of the words are meaningful communications...instead they are just noise? Or has life just become so vindictive that it is impossible to trust (and this heart / throat chakra medicine is discussed at length in *The Aromatherapy Bronchitis Treatment*)

Just for ease, I am copying out of The Mind Body Spirit of Essential Oils so you can get an easy reference to the chakra medicine. I also feel that the sacral chakra and its effects on one's own "self perception" has a bearing here too.

Throat

Located: As one would expect

Aligned to: Communication, expression, truth

Vibrates on the colour: Blue

By the time we get to the throat chakra we starting to find ways we can express what we want from life. We begin to explore how we can manifest the reality we desire. A balanced throat chakra makes our voice clear and bright, our words are resilient and come out just right. But if the energy is off, we can find words come out garbled or intelligible to hear. Our words can often stick and struggle to make it out to others ears.

Not just words though, it is any kind of expression. Working in the throat chakra can mean your water colour painting improves or even the way you dance. One thing I have noticed, when my throat chakra is off, is my rhythm and timing also goes awry.

The reason for this strange phenomenon might have something to do with the way the throat chakra melds the head and the heart. It is the seat of integrity. Do the words the mouth says reflect an accord between the heart and the head? Lying for example, does not. Swallowing your pride does not. Delivering news for the good of the company at the expense of the people does not. Perhaps then, the off-rhythm is that tiny little beat we miss as we check our truths.

So what ways might this manifest? Coughing, sore throats, starting to mumble, jitter, or even developing a stammer for some, are all classic indicators that something with the throat chakra might be amiss.

Problems with not expressing your truths through the throat chakra might lead to physical disturbances such as:

Sore throats and other disorders in the upper respiratory tract, ear problems (think: *no, I'm sorry, I just don't want to hear!*) problems with the oesophagus and also the cervical neck and spine. (*Think: I've had a gut full of this and it's all becoming a bit of a pain in the neck!*) In extreme cases these problems might also cause issues with the thyroid gland and the hypothalamus. In less acute cases you may find a fever also comes with throat problems, almost as if to purge.

How strange that the chakra connected with expression has the most obvious spoken clues!

Sacral

Located: 2 ins below the navel

Is aligned to: Abundance, well being, pleasure and sexuality

Vibrates on the colour: Orange

So as we start to grow, then our spiritual awareness lifts up. This is the energy of the older child, not quite adolescent. It is about creativity, the birth of sexuality, control and again, money. Here though, think of all of these in the context of one's own individuality.

Blockages of this energy will be seen as what we might dismissively call playground tactics but of course, uncomfortable as it is to admit, very few of us actually grow out of them.

Think:

- Power plays

- Jealousy or envy
- Betrayal
- Control

Physical disturbances you might see associated with sacral chakra energy are:

Sexual problems, in particular, impotence and frigidity, problems with the bladder and urinary tracts, and also issues in the large intestine.

Here, I think it is worth commenting on the chicken and egg situation between emotions and the chakras. Sometimes the depleted energy will lead to a specific emotion, in this case let's say playing power games. But, just as often, the emotion will mess with the chakra energy too. A person betrayed, may try to exert control and probably won't want to have sex. The chakra didn't cause the physical issue....it carried it. There is always this constant fluctuation and communication between the three, always interlocked and potentially all showing problems in one way or another...no one single catalyst.

Chapter 3 - The Medicinal Uses of Basil

Basil in Aromatherapy

There are many chemotypes of Sweet Basilavailable on the market. It will become clear when you get to the clinical data why I now opt for "Basil linalool" because of its marked effects on the emotional body, but there are many people selling a methyl chavicol chemotype too. Methyl chavicol is also known as euganol. Whilst not carcinogenic in its own right, it is a precursor to some metabolites which are believed might be. Its fragrance is different to linalool chemotype in that it has a delicious anise fragrance, so it is popular in perfumery but also for blending diffuser mixes and incenses. It is not recommended for long term general usage because of these concerns.

Extraction
Steam distillation from flowering tops and leaves

Main constituents
Linalool, methyl chavicol, euganol, limonene, citronella

Properties
- Anti depressant

- Antiseptic

- Antispasmodic

- Carminative

- Cephalic (Clears the brain)

- Diuretic

- Emmenagoguic (stimulates blood flow to the pelvis – often to stimulate menstruation)

- Expectorant (Gets rid of phlegm)

- Febrifigal (Reduces fever)

- Galactagoguic (Increases breast milk)* see end of list

- Hepatic (only slightly so, but nevertheless)

- Protective to the kidneys

- Intestinal antiseptic

- Nervine (For the nerves!)

- Prophylactic (Preventing disease)

- Restorative

- Stimulant of the adrenal cortex

- Stomachic

- Tonic

Most of these are covered in their own way in different parts of the book so I am not going to labour by repeating. Here are some snippets that are not.

Breast Milk

I am going to start with the breast milk because I am not happy with this one. I think the strong taste of the oil and the methyl chavicol content (in all chemotypes) makes it a poorer choice than geranium, celery and carrot.

Emmenagogue

I thought I would just bring you a lovely account from John Parkinson's work where he discusses how to use Basil to bring on menstruation. Clearly he used herbs, you can use oil. Drop into hot water and place the bowl under a slotted chair. The woman should sit astride the chair devoid of underwear for twenty minutes then lie down with her legs raised and cover herself with a blanket.

Aromatherapy from the bottom up!

Expectorant

My experience of this is that inhalation tends to work better than topical administration, but because I am always nervous of the decision, I tend to do it both ways! Basil is an extremely good oil for the respiratory system and should be one of the first ones you buy for coughs and colds because catarrh and phlegm doesn't stand a chance against it.

Prophylactic

(Titter titter – that's what I can remember my mum calling condoms when I was kid! I was very confused and had to look it up and now the fact that it means "preventing disease" makes sense). Here, the prophylactic action probably comes from its antioxidant properties and also on its affects on the adrenals inhibiting stress related inflammation.

Aromatherapy Uses

- Muscular aches and pains
- Respiratory disorders
- Scant menstruation
- Colds and influenza
- Chest infections, in particular bronchitis and emphysema
- Gastric spasm
- Dyspepsia
- Coughs and in particular whooping cough (Valnet)
- Malaria(both symptoms and also as insect repellent)
- Migraine
- Epilepsy
- Jaundice (Davis)
- Paralysis (Valnet)

- Gout
- Nervous debility
- Nervous insomnia
- Mental fatigue
- Anxiety
- Depression
- Loss of smell due to catarrh
- Wasp stings, scorpion stings, snake bite (First aid whilst the ambulance is on its way)
- Mouth wash for ulcers

Safety concerns

This is very strong oil and can irritate the skin and so I would recommend using in dilutions of less than 1%.

Do not use in pregnancy.

Basil in Chinese Medicine

Luo Le (Sweet Basil herb)

Properties

Pungent, sweet, warm;

Tonic to the lung, spleen, stomach and large intestine meridians

Actions

Basil dispels wind and promotes the flow of qi. It eliminates dampness and promotes better digestion. It activates the blood and it remove toxicity.

Uses

- Irregular menstruation

- Itchy eyes*

- Abdominal cramps

- Eczema*

- Snake and insect bites

- Traumatic injury

- Diarrhoea

- Indigestion

- Urticaria*

- Headache

* There seems to be a great deal of usage of Basil for itchiness of various types in TCM, which we would not see in aromatherapy. This is interesting to me. I wonder if this is an action that can only be found from the whole plant and does not pass through to distillation.

Dosage and administration

Here Basil is used as a decoction using between 5~15 g of leaves, boiled for 20 minutes and then left to cool to drink or more often used as a cooling liquid to be used externally.

Sometimes the leaves are pounded to make juice, or they made be made into pills and powder. Proper dosage is for external application, pounded for applying, or decocted for washing or mouthwash.

Cautions

It is contraindicated in case of qi deficiency, where vitality is low because of long term stress, malnutrition, old age, weak constitution. (Typical Basil contradiction, this would seem at surface level to be the opposite of aromatherapy usage!)

Each organ has their own manifestation of qi deficiency. Here are some symptoms you might want to look for.

Lung

- Breathlessness
- Weak Voice
- Spontaneous Sweating

Spleen

- Loss of Appetite

- Loose Stools

- Fatigue

- Normal or Pale and Swollen Tongue

Heart

- Palpitations

Kidney

- Frequent Urination

- Possible Lower Back Pain and Weak Knees

- Possible Poor Memory

Basil in Ayurveda

Ayurveda was the first of the holistic medical regimes and gives us our first insight into how Basil aligns the mind body and spirit. Ayurvedic medicine seeks to bring the outer body: the skin, hair, nails, into alignment with the inner body which is clearly all the internal processing organs, digestive, respiratory etc, but also thoughts and feelings too. When the inner body and outer body are in accord, then the radiant secret shines forth.

In order to achieve this, they work on a framework of doshas and how an excess of one will send the whole system out of balance. At the point of conception we gain pakruti, which is our inherent disposition towards a certain type. I for instance am most definitely pitta – kapha, where my husband is kapha pitta. They do say opposites attract!

The Basil **_plant and oil_** suppress vata and kapha. The _seeds_ however are suppressant to pitta and kapha. It is a good anti inflammatory and pain reliever. It is potent and hot. Because it a very light oil it is excellent for digestive issues. It stimulates the heart and purifies the blood. It relieves burning in the body and is aphrodisiac.

Vata
Vata is the connection between air and ether. It governs movement. It oversees the nervous system and the elimination systems of the body.

Those of you who have read my vetiver book will recognise the next few paragraphs of explanation of vata and kapha.

Words which describe vata are:

98

Light, cold, dry, rough, changeable, moving, and quick

The vata physical frame is thin, light and slender.

Their energy is quick and comes in very short bursts. They can be prone to fatigue.

Basil is very good at "undoing" this burnout.

They will feel the cold severely and their connective tissue, their skin, hair and teeth are dry and brittle. Their sleep is very light and the digestion is changeable.

Basil improves digestion and in cases of insomnia from adrenal fatigue will bring the central nervous system back into alignment to help them to sleep.

When vata is unbalanced there is often weight loss, trouble sleeping, irritability, and joint problems such as arthritis.

I would agree that Basil would be the oil of choice in all these cases.

Emotionally, vatas love new experiences and they bore very easily. Their tempers ignite very quickly, but also forgive at the same speed. When their energy is in balance they are wonderfully creative, happy to take initiatives in new ideas. They are eloquent conversationalists and are deliciously flexible people to be around; they are happy to go with the flow. What you will find though, is they are thinkers rather than doers and tend to be more interested in theories rather than practical applications of things.

From the discoveries we made in the spiritual realm, we know now, that these *balanced* aspects of a person's personality would lead you *away* from Basil. There will be better oils to use. But if you strive to *engender* these to heal a person, especially on an emotional or spiritual dimension, then this might be the oil to consider.

When out of balance though vata energy makes worriers and these people in particular can really suffer from insomnia.

Absolutely, **this is Basil medicine.**

Kapha

To recap: Basil oil suppresses kapha, so it will push that energy down.

The primary function of kapha is protection and it governs the connective tissues of the body, the bones, muscles, fat and sinews

Words to describe kapha are:

Heavy, slow, soft, oily, steady, solid, careful

Kapha are the big guys and gals. They have big builds and huge amounts of stamina. They have lovely soft eyes and almost oily sheens to their skins. They have thick and lustrous hair.

Emotionally they are steady people, completely reliable and very calm. They are thoughtful and loving and they are most comfortable with a steady routine. Emotional imbalance of kapha, though, will lead to stubbornness and burying their heads in the sand. Of all the doshas this one is the most resistant to change with these people staying in jobs and relationships long after they have outgrown them.

Here, Basil will shake the foundations of the world to the core. Basil likes stability and predictability if this is correct for the spirit, but if a person is protecting the status quo and ignoring the spiritual messages they should be hearing then Basil will make some changes.

When kapha is in balance they are good sleepers and have excellent digestion but when kapha builds, the digestion becomes more sluggish and the sleep seems to go on and on. They simply get slower and slower and harder to move! Often these people can suffer from diabetes, asthma and depression.

Digestion is of foremost importance here, and Basil is especially useful for treating constipation in particular. Later though, in the clinical trials, you will be

dumbfounded by the wisdom lasting over 5000 years, of Basil for diabetes, asthma and depression – especially depression.

For completeness, I am adding pitta in here, because the seeds suppress it. But remember the oil does not really have a bearing here and actually this is useful to see when basil would be a bad choice. You'll notice that the pitta temperament is very similar to the oil itself so we don't want to inflame "the condition" any more.

Pitta
Words to describe pitta:

Hot, oily, fiery, sharp, inflamed, intense, penetrating, pungent

Physically pittas are usually of fairly average size and weight. Many have bright red hair (remind you of anyone?), but you will often see their hair as thinning or balding too. They have the constitutions of an ox so they will believe they can eat anything and everything in the house. They have massive appetites and good enough digestion to deal with that.

See? No requirement for Basil.

Their body temperature is warm. They have lustrous complexions with an almost oily sheen to it. Problems start when their pitta energy goes out of balance and they will suffer from sensitive skins and rashes. Their internal and external heating goes out of control leading to hot inflamed skins, burning cystitis or hot flushes. The first sign of the pitta imbalance will come when their digestion decides it has had enough and they start complaining of heartburn, and indigestion.

Again, we don't want to heat the situation any more, we want to cool it.

Pittas are very sharp witted and often can be a tad too outspoken and direct in their opinions. Because they are extremely concise they make excellent teachers and public speakers. They can concentrate very well and have very powerful intellects which make them clear, astute decision makers.

On a bad day they are short tempered and extremely argumentative. (I am so not!!!)

Basil can create enough trouble on her own, without adding an already fiery temperament into the mix.

Just as the wind can move the earth, as sand across the desert, and ripples across the water, so vata controls and dominates the other doshas. In other words it is going to be the vata personality traits you see manifesting that will drive the physical and emotional complaints of the other doshas.

To make that simpler, let's turn the vata description into a negative so you can see traits you are looking for:

Emotionally, vatas love new experiences and they bore very easily.

- Look for a resistance to change and an unhealthy comfort with routine (Is it like a safety blanket preventing them from taking risks for instance?)
- Or the other side of the coin: are they flighty and non committal to an unhealthy degree

Their tempers ignite very quickly, but also forgive at the same speed.

- Unforgiving and point scoring
- Forgiving bad behaviour far too easily and often (for example in a domestic violence situation)
- Making excuses for someone's behaviour – and that might actually be their own
- Don't get angry enough. No passion. No rage.
- Far too volatile

When their energy is in balance they are wonderfully creative, happy to take initiatives in new ideas.

- Extension of the first point, really.

They are eloquent conversationalists and are deliciously flexible people to be around; they are happy to go with the flow.

- Hog the conversation so no-one else can get a word in

- Do not allow other people to speak

- Dogmatic

- Controlling

- Lacking in flexibility overly rigid in their thinking

- Do not speak up for themselves

- Being too flexible, letting other people control them

I'd expect to see "spineless" in some people hereWhat you will find though, is they are thinkers rather than doers and tend to be more interested in theories rather than practical applications of things.

- So you might see people who never execute an idea or action, it all stays in their head
- An excess of vata is most definitely "acting out" and never engaging the brain before the mouth or fists.

Chapter 4 Basil Essential Oil

Botany

Family: Lamiaceae

This is the same family of aromatic plants that lavenders and mints (amongst others) hail from. You might also sometimes see it listed as St Joseph's Wort in some herbals. It has a characteristic square, hairy stem, *labiate* flowers which have the characteristic appearance of lips, and also opposite leaves. It has a rich, spicy aroma reminiscent of mints, cloves and pepper.

The Ocimum family is vast with around 160 different cultivars available on the market. Most notable of these is Holy Basil which is sacred to the Hindus, and is the subject of another one of my books. Often you will see them linked together in internet write-ups but on closer examination they are as different as chalk and jelly fish! There is probably only one thing that botanists and herbalists are in agreement about and that is that Basil loves the sun and heat above all other things.

Pliny wrote testimony to cursing when sowing Basil seeds, and went on to explain that they should be sown on April 21st at the feast of Pales. Then, when the Dog Star rises, Basil turns pale. Here we have a glance into a time when the calendar was entirely different to our own. To the Greeks and Romans, The Dog-Days when Sirius rode high in the sky were the reason for the sun's ferocious heat. Between July 3rd to August 11th, Sirius rises in conjunction with the sun. It was believed that the brightest star of day (the sun) and the brightest star of night (the Dog Star) joined together to fiercely heat the earth.

In Egypt, the coming of the Dog Days was prepared for by the priests, at the Feast of Isis. For Sirius is the star of Isis and when she rose high in the sky there would be madness, droughts and plagues. The priests were the calendar keepers of Egypt and they would watch for Sirius rising just moments before the sun. An aisle lined by tall columns ran through the temple of Isis-Hathor at Denderah. At the end was a statue of the goddess. A jewel was placed in the goddess' forehead.

The statue was turned to the rising of Sirius, so that the light from the returning Dog Star would spark upon the gem casting rays around the room. On that first glimmer, the priests would march from the temple and announce the beginning of their New Year. An inscription appears on the walls of the temple: "Her majesty Isis shines into the temple on New Year's Day, and she mingles her light with that of her father Ra on the horizon."

So much more in tune with their (flat) planet, than we ever can be, I think, now, the Ancient Egyptians knew that the rising of Sirius would also bring the rising of the Nile in the next few days. They prepared to open the floodgate to bring fertility to their lands with her swell. The canals gates were opened and the thirsty lands of Egypt prepared for a well deserved drink.

A busy time, I would have thought, and in that seasonal frenzy the gardeners would be very mindful it was also time to harvest one's Basil....

Strangely marking the passage of time, 5000 years ago this would have happened on June 25th. In 2015, our calendars show Sirius rising in August. In ancient articles, you will see Sirius described as the Sparkling One (since she shows as pale blue in the sky and can sometimes be seen with her radiance splitting like a rainbow) or The Scorching One. I think in the context of Basil the latter fits her better.

Usually when we are looking for Roman usages of herbs, Theophastrus will furnish us with wonderful data, but here, in his Enquiry of Plants we see Basil being treated very carefully again. He does not speak of any medicinal or culinary usage only that it grows differently from other plants. Sown in April, where other plants have one big floral show Theophastrus notices that Basil works differently with flowers starting at the base of the stem and working their way up. *(Is it just me or does that feel sinewy and snake like to you too?)* The flowers appear as a whorl in summer and are usually white or pale pink or purple.

The chemistry of Basil changes radically after it has flowered. The scent and flavour both become bitterer. When growing Basil it is preferable to keep removing the tops to prevent the flowers from forming and to prolong Basil's "year".

The chemistry also changes from fresh leaf to dry. When left, the leaves form a greater strength of euganol which as described in the chemistry section, is a precursor to a metabolite thought to be carcinogenic. For this reason dried herb consumption should be limited (not enough concern to say eradicated) but fresh leaves are preferable.

Sixteenth century botanist Bauhin announced "the contrariness of Basil" in that, unlike any other plant he can think of she "wants to be watered in the heat of the day". His contemporary, Italian botanist, André Matolli considered that the original name Ocymum may have come from the Greek *Ocys* meaning swift growing.

Costaeus (16th Century), ponders about the feebleness of the plant, and how it will wither if it does not get regular attention and watering. He concludes that basil must have a laxity of substance which causes its innate heat to be easily disrupted, meaning it requires a continual source of heat to support its constant need for nourishment.

Heat – drama- constant attention – narcissism....

Round and round the healing goes...where will it stop...?

Nobody knows.

Chemistry

Chemical composition of Basil extracts reveals the presences of tanines, flavonoids, saponins, and volatile terpenes like camphor, tymol, methylchavicol, linalool, eugenol, 1-8-cineol and pinenes.

The Basil plant is not very good at keeping secrets about its yield and a moment's research of the pollen under a microscope discloses the potential for essential oil production each plant has. Three striations (stripes) across a granule of pollen shows a density of sesquiterpenes, but the essential oil yield will be low. Six striations, however, shows a plant high in monoterpenols, or alcohols, and which will also will give a far greater yield of oil. Later, when we get to the clinical trials you will see that the

110

chemotypes with a higher potential of linalol (those with 6 striations) are the most useful to us, especially in the treatment of inflammation and depression.

You might see some chemotypes of oil marked as Ocimum Basilicum var. "European" this is the Lettuce Leaf Basil. Here the levels of methyl chavicol plummet to 10-15% (from the more usual 50%) and the levels of linalool rockets to about 40% of the oil's constituency

The majority of the Basil oils you will find on the market are high in methyl chavicol and this gives the oil a more liquorice-y / aniseed note.

Note
Middle

Blends well with
Bergamot, black pepper, cedarwood, citronella, clary sage, fennel, frankincense, geranium, ginger, grapefruit, hyssop, lavender, lemon verbena, lime, marjoram, neroli, oakmoss, rose.

Most green note herbs will work too, coriander, parsley etc. etc.

If we look to the ancient laws of alchemy we find that Venus tempers Mars. In fact Culpepper, himself, alluded to it at the beginning of the book *"and as it helps the deficiency of Venus in one kind, so it spoils all her actions in another.*

In other words, Venus balances Mars. Sometimes she will make him work harder, others not so much.

Now we start to see the beauty of the plant medicine.

Venus is the ruler of rose.

Put a Victorian young lady, the typical English rose, next to our Italian Basil girl. The stereotypes give the magic away. The cool detached romance of the rose next to the spicy hotness of the Mediterranean, exciting, sexy, unpredictable...

No wonder Rose and Basil work so magically together in blends! They support each other and they balance each other out. I can almost see rose's gentle hand extending through time to reach the trauma and gently help it through the door that Basil kicked so rudely open.

Not all of these plants have essential oils, but since many healers use plants to make flower essences, tinctures, etc.

And meld these into their aromatherapy, I have chosen to list all botanicals for a more rounded view.

Many flowers come under Venus if they are particularly beautiful to look at, so you might also consider jonquil, hyacinth or neroli for instance:

- Benzoin
- Cardamom
- Cistus / Labdanum
- Daffodil
- Golden rod
- Honey suckle
- Jasmine
- Lilac
- Lily
- Mint
- Myrtle
- Palma rosa
- Rose
- Rose geranium
- Sage
- Sandalwood
- Spearmint
- Thyme

- Tonka

- Valerian

- Vanilla

- Vervain

- Violet

- Ylang-ylang

- Yarrow

- Most spices

Safety Data

The following data is taken from *Essential Oil Safety Tisserand and Young (2013)*. In my opinion, anyone using essential oils on a regular basis should own a copy. It is fascinating to compare the different chemotypes of oils, but also the library of scientific data in this book exceeds even mine. The book's lists of active constituents are far more in depth than I will give you here, but I shall list the two primary constituents in each. Based on our findings throughout the book this should enable you have more clarity about which Basil oil will help you best when you order new supplies

Three things of note before we start:

You will find chemotypes and sister subspecies that are not mentioned elsewhere in the book. This is purely because I found them interesting for comparison, no other.

Secondly, there is little parity between the sources of the recommendations of safe limits of use. I am going to add to that confusion and further worsen it, I'm afraid. Remember *their* details, that is IFRA (International Fragrance Association) and those of Tisserand and Young, are based on the amount of the oil used on a rat (probably) before it developed a rash or some kind of internal organ damage. I shall base *mine* on how much is safe before scorpions grow in your brain...or at least you start to be more Martian than you should be!

Based on how strong the emotional energy of the oil is, and the fact that Basil *can* be skin sensitising, I would agree with Julia Lawless...not more than 1% and she goes as far as to say probably err on the side of inhalation rather than topical use. I think she is right about that, but I shall still continue to use topically, just less regularly than oils such as say...geranium, for instance. Lastly, I am going to suggest different safety data entirely for pregnancy. That is:

Do not use Basil in the first 16 weeks of pregnancy and if used later please use in dilutions of 0.5%.

I think you will find it interesting to see just how different the chemistry of oils from one species can be.

Hoary Basil (aka. Hairy Basil)
Ocimum americanum L. Var pilosum (Wild)

Linalol 31.7-50.1%

Estragol 0.3-0.4%

Maximum dermal limit according to:

- IFRA 2.5%
- Tisserand and Young 30%
- Secret Healer 1%

Lemon Basil
Ocimum x citriodorum vis

Geranial 23.3-25.1%

Neral 16.0-17.1%

Nerol 13.0-15.3%

Linalool 5.0-7.8%

Maximum dermal limit according to:

- IFRA 1.4%
- Tisserand and Young 1.4%
- Secret Healer 1%

Contraindications: Affects diabetes meds and should not be used at any stage of pregnancy.

Basil Linalool CT
Ocimum Basilicum L

Linalool 34.4%

Euganol 33.7%

Maximum dermal limit according to:

- IFRA 1.5%
- Tisserand and Young 1.5%
- Secret Healer 1%

Contraindications: None listed

Basil Methyl cinnamate CCT

Ocimum Basilicum L

Methyl cinnamate 58.0-63.1

Linalool 17.3-27.3

Maximum dermal limit according to:

- IFRA 1.5%
- Tisserand and Young 15%
- Secret Healer 1%

Contraindications: None listed

Basil Pungent

Ocimum gratissimum

Euganol 62.7%

(E) β- ocimene 20.6

Maximum dermal limit according to:

- IFRA 0.1%
- Tisserand and Young 4.6%
- Secret Healer 1%

Contraindications: Affects pethedine and anticoagulant medications such as warfarin, heparin or enoxoparin. Do not use with a bleeding disorder such as haemophilia or a bleeding ulcer.

You might find it interesting to compare these with Holy Basil in my other book.

Where to Buy your Basil Oils

I have been getting more and more email lately asking for recommendations on oils suppliers, and it has been a theme running through some of the reviews of my books.

Oshadhi are my essential oils supplier of choice. They have a range of nearly 500 oils, in particular ones harder to find in mainstream stores. The quality of their oils is exquisite, as they choose to deal with more artisan producers and companies that distil their oils more slowly.

Often companies may distil for four hours, for example to produce more products in a day, but this slower distillation, for perhaps 6 hours allows time for the larger molecules to come through. These are richer, deeper scented molecules. The difference between these and standard commercial essential oils is easily discernible by scent, but the difference also passes through to its superior therapeutic uses too.

Oshadhi's website can be found at (UK)

http://www.oshadhi.co.uk/

http://www.oshadhi.com/ (US)

Chapter 5 Clinical Evidence of Basil's Healing Prowess

It is hard to know where to start with this part. Even more so than others of my books there is a spider's web of interactions with the medicine and how they all interlock.

I think I we'll start with Basil's anti-inflammatory actions.

Anti- Inflammatory

Recent psychoneuroendocrinological studies show that **inflammation in the body is directly related to hostility we feel**. In particular, studies into the correlation between abuse (mental/ physical/sexual) in childhood resoundingly predict the probability of chronic disease in adulthood. I wrote about this at length in my book The Aromatherapy Bronchitis Treatment because a person who has a high emotional impact score can be as much as three times as likely to develop COPD.

I am adding a link here to a summary of Adverse Children's Experience Study for you.

http://acestudy.org/files/Review_of_ACE_Study_with_r eferences_summary_table_2_.pdf

There are some very controversial arguments that suggest poorly understood syndromes like Chronic Pelvic Pain Syndrome, Chronic Fatigue Syndrome, Fibromyalgia and

Irritable Bowel Syndrome might, in fact, be one and the same. That these illnesses which seem to have no physical explanation, but seem to be triggered and exacerbated by stress, might all be different manifestations of the body's response to some degree of trauma. As if the body is saying the same thing, in different languages, if you like. (Incidentally the jury is still deliberating on this and I can see they will be out for many years more. I think the argument has aspects that are compelling but I still have a way to go before I am wholly convinced.)

To the untrained ear, the phrase "put it down to stress" might seem patronising and derogatory but this is anything but. Anyone who suffered at the hands of an anxiety led response knows just how like a puppet you can feel. There is an overwhelming feeling that one must control the stress and that becomes another stress factor on top...and the symptoms simply get worse.

If we were to see the notes the doctor had written about our consultation we might find the word *somatic / somatisation/ somatising*. I talk about this extensively in my book *Sales Strategies For Gentle Souls* because it is the area of illness where there seems to be no physical explanation for illness and doctors suppose that perhaps it may be purely emotional. Remember these *soma* words, as in *psychosomatic,* as they will serve your understanding well later on.

Many of you will know there are three driving directions of my research. The first is blood, because I suffered a blood clot in my lungs, which also leads me to the second area- the respiratory system. A lesser known area is Chronic Pelvic Pain Syndrome (CPP) after having reduced a patient's symptoms in a week where many doctors had been perplexed and stumped for years. The healing surprised me more than anyone, especially since there were 43 oils in the blend. There are still many pieces that must be found to this particular jigsaw puzzle, but of all the work I have done with patients so far, this is the one of which I am the most proud.

Over the subsequent years I have become fascinated by the work done by Rita Valentino and her research into CRF1. This molecule, Cortisone Releasing Factor was first introduced to me in Candace Pert's work where she described it as the **Molecule of Negative Expectation.** Sadly, part of that name had arisen because it is found in almost ten times the volume of the spinal cords of people who have committed suicide.

Valentino went on to demonstrate that the Nucleus of Barrington, a part of the brain also sometime referred to as the pons, was filled with receptors for the molecule. This area of the brain is fundamentally involved with micturation, or as the rest of us would say "going for a wee!" This fascinated me and it made me think of my patient, one of whose problems with CPP was visiting the bathroom to urinate as many as 20 times in a day, but only passing tiny volumes of water.

It is a fairly well accepted assumption, now, that CPP probably results from sort of conditioned trauma, presenting in pelvic pain during micturation, excretion, exercise and sex, including the arousal stage as well as penetration and climax... The overwhelming numbers of Gulf War veterans (both male and female) living with this pain is testament to this. So what if, I wondered, the key to relieving the pain lived in eradicating the effects of the trauma through the tissues?

My own patient was not a soldier, but instead a woman who had suffered at the hands of a cruel manipulator. He had been emotionally and physically violent and although she did not know for sure whether he had been unfaithful, she felt that it would have been outside of his nature not to be.

To my mind Basil help her take back control. Not just of her emotions but her bladder too. In just one day her urine output went from 2 fl oz in a visit to the toilet to 6 fl oz to nearly 12 fl oz. A healthy bladder should be able to retain about a pint become it needs to vacate. The previous day she had counted 15 visits to the ladies room, after treatment, he counted just six. After one period cycle pain was completely vanished.

Incidentally, the role of the Nucleus of Barrington is only to force the bladder to contract. By contrast in 2005, researchers at University of Tokyo were able to discern that while the nucleus excites the bladder, it plays no part in the bladders relaxation. So what if Dioscorides had had the answer all along? **Basil helps those with difficulty in urination (through its diuretic action).** But my mind, like the butterfly it can be, refuses to rest with that because I think it goes further in that Basil is also a tonic for the kidneys. In Chinese Medicine the kidneys govern fear. What if Basil released the grip of that fear and allowed the bladder to relax and let go?

We know too, that one of the primary protagonists of inflammation in the body is Interleukin- 6. This pro-inflammatory cytokine is the source of great discussion, for obvious reasons, and in 2013 a paper was published by the University of Cork (Ireland) entitled *Crosstalk between interleukin-6 and corticotropin-releasing factor modulate submucosal plexus activity and colonic secretion*. Here they were interested in the neurotransmitter conversations that might be in play when a person suffers from IBS. Here at least some of my thoughts were confirmed that this molecule of negative emotion seemed to affect the inflammatory chemistry and, in turn, this switched on the pain and discomfort of the gastric symptoms.

http://www.ncbi.nlm.nih.gov/pubmed/23369733

Similar findings here: http://onlinelibrary.wiley.com/doi/10.1113/jphysiol.2014.279968/abstract

And through a more complex explanation here:

http://joe.endocrinology-journals.org/content/195/2/199.full.pdf

Of all the research I can find on *Ocimum Basilicum*, the most important ones, to me, seem to be into fibromyalgia and also as an anti-depressant. Let's start with fibromyalgia because I seem to hear of this condition more and more.

A Brazilian team in December 2014 released the details of a series of experiments they had undertaken on some Swiss mice. The white furry scamperers had had hyperalgesia chemically induced. What this term pertains to is **an increased sensitivity to pain**. Fibromyalgia is a chronic musculoskeletal disorder characterized by chronic widespread pain, presence of tender points on physical examination, as well as symptoms that include fatigue, morning stiffness, sleep disorders and depression. Sadly, we still do not know why it happens and as previously mentioned there are those who class it as a non-disease. Clearly that is an orthodox medicinal term, since we as complementary therapists would argue that a sufferer is clearly *not* at ease with this condition and so decidedly *is* dis-eased.

The main argument with fibromyalgia is between two rooms of psychological experts. The first say fibromyalgia is a manifestation of depression. Their argument has support from the fact that many people's symptoms improve through anti depressant drugs and also cognitive behavioural therapy and counselling.

The second school of thought says, no. That's not right. That depression might often happen *because* of the pain, or it might happen *as well* as the muscle fatigue, migraines and pain etc, but they don't happen *because* of it. There has been some recent research that has discovered that patients with the condition seem to have small areas between muscle fibres that lack a myelin sheath the protect them. This myelin sheath is made of proteins that act like an insulator taking messages from the muscles to the brain. Without this protective layer, the nerves are more exposed to external stimulus. This, in turn, adds weight to *their* argument.

I think as complimentary therapists we have a distinct advantage here, in that our holistic treatment requires we look at the whole person rather than breaking it down and so, really, all we need to know is the patient hurts emotionally and physically. There is no need for us to strip these down...especially when Basil results show it **alleviates this hyperalgesia and also depression.**

Our red eyed, little white furry friends were able to reveal some fascinating data. It was found that *Ocimum Basilicum* was able to block nociceptive receptors. These are the receptors that send messages via the spinal column to the brain about potentially damaging substances. In other words **these receptors give us our *perception* of pain.**

The poor rodents were injected with a substance into their calf muscle to trigger discomfort. Gradually day by day el-mousey put less and less weight on it until the 27th day when his responses were tested. (I should think the poor thing was fixing the scientist firmly with his little red eyes picturing right where he's like to stuff his Swiss Army Knife by day 26!) This day 27 reading was compared with giving our furry friend a blitz of Basil an hour before his test on the 28th day. Here, on day 28 mucho-relieved Mickey withdrew his paw less, because of this nociceptive response. In other words he wasn't so afraid of the pain he would feel when he put it down.

In the fibromyalgia syndrome, it is thought that areas of tissue insulated with myelin tends to react in the same way as parts of the body where there is no myelin protection, leading the sufferer to have a more acute experience of pain, even from the very lightest of pressures.

Recent data showed that (−)-linalool, the major compound of Sweet Basil oil, blocks this myelin pain in a concentration-dependent and reversible manner. For us as aromatherapists this is a massive breakthrough, because we know that a drop of Basil in our massage blends should be very helpful, but for the drug companies this is not enough. The fact that oils do not mix with water makes them very difficult to make into commercial drugs to help the masses. The half life too, is a complication. This is the time it takes for a substance's concentration to reduce by half and so eventually be absent from the blood plasma. The half life of an essential oil is very quick. So then, they must look for secondary metabolites in the oil that they might be able to synthesize to replicate the effects. Here we find that β-Cyclodextrin-complexed –(-) linalool will be their avenue of choice.

Most importantly from this trial we see a shining beacon in New Paradigm medicine. The author relates that *"The synergistic effect of (−)-linalool exerts modulatory effect of pain through central and peripheral mechanisms can provide benefits for the management of chronic pain syndromes such as fibromyalgia because it acts by different mechanisms and it can activate different pathways of the central nervous system.*

Nerves...physical nerves, but an unmistakable connection to emotional ones too.

Now, the dose dependant claim about the Basil is the most interesting aspect of this trial because it is counterintuitive. I groaned when I read it and rubbed my head because I thought it meant that you needed *more and more* Basil for it to work, and that goes against everything I have discovered so far, but I should be more patient with myself!

The research details; and I quote:

"The variability in the 100mg/kg treatment [shown in figure 3] suggests a probable phenomenon called hormeosis. This paradoxical effect has been observed n a great number of organisms, and with a large number of poisons and drugs

Hormeosis?

Well, the word comes from ancient Greek stem word that translates to "rapid motion, eagerness". It means it works more potently the less you use! (Just look over to the door for a sec, Mars is winking at you. Give him a wave!)

Now, research into Basil is not new and there is now quite a lot of understanding into the pathways that – (-) linalool pathways activate. It is believed that it modulates the following channels:

- Opioid
- Dopinergic
- Adrenergic
- Muscarinic
- Glutamatergic

Just as a quick rundown in case we have gone too scientific

Opioid
Resembling opium in its pain relieving and addictive effects. Found in the brain, but also in the spinal cord and digestive tracts. There are many types of Opioid receptors, you will now recognise nociceptor from our poor Swiss mice. (When you see what these receptors can do it's a good job Mickey didn't have a weapon stashed!)

There are four types of Opioid receptors:

delta (δ) DOR
Areas of the brain these are found in are:

pontine nuclei (remember our bladder?) amygdala, olfactory bulbs, deep cortex

And in the peripheral sensory systems:

neurons

The functions of this group of receptors are:

- analgesia

- antidepressant effects

- convulsant effects

- physical dependence (being dependent on a substance that you develop a tolerance but withdrawal would cause adverse symptoms)

- may modulate μ-opioid receptor-mediated respiratory depression

kappa (κ)- KOR
Areas of the brain these are found in are:

Hypothalamus, periaqueductal gray, claustrum,

They are also found in the spinal cord in the substantia gelatinosa peripheral and also in neurons.

Functions of this group of receptors are:

- analgesia

- anticonvulsant effects

- depression

- dissociative/hallucinogenic effects

- dieresis (kidneys produce urine)

- dysphoria (feelings of dissatisfaction in life)

- miosis (constricts the pupils)

- neuroprotection

- sedation

- stress

mu (μ) MOR

Areas of the brain these are found in are:

Cortex, thalamus, striosomes, periaqueductal gray, rostral ventromedial medulla

Also found in the spinal cord in the substantia gelatinosa

As well as in sensory neurons as well as the intestinal tract.

Functions of this group of receptors are:

- analgesia

- physical dependence

- respiratory depression

- miosis

- euphoria

- reduced GI motility (stomach problems)

- physical dependence

- possible vasodilation

Nociceptin receptors - NOP

Areas of the brain these are found in are:

Cortex, amygdala, hippocampus, septal nuclei, habenula

hypothalamus

They are also found in the spinal cord.

Functions of this group of receptors are:

- anxiety

- depression

- appetite

Dopamine

The dopamine receptors in the body are involved in many aspects of our emotional well being as well as some physical aspects. Functions include motivation, pleasure, cognition, memory and learning. Most notably dopamine modulates neuroendocrine signalling, that is to say they bring together the messaging between the nervous system and the endocrine system.

Because abnormal dopamine receptor signalling and dopaminergic nerve function is implicated in several neuropsychiatric disorders, dopamine receptors are common neurologic drug targets; antipsychotics drugs are often created from dopamine receptor antagonists.

Adrenergic

This denotes nerve cells where adrenaline, noradrenalin, as well as other similar substances, act as neurotransmitters. These are directly connected to the adrenal system and are fundamentally attached to stress related (and by extension *somatic*) responses. This area is explained in more depth in *The Professional Stress Solution*.

Muscarinic

Muscarinic receptors trigger *acetylcholine*, a neurotransmitter in the autonomic nervous system. It acts on both the peripheral nervous system and central nervous system. It is the only neurotransmitter that plays a part in the motor division (ie physical dimension) of the **somatic** nervous system.

Glutamatergic

This family of receptors exists in the greatest number in the brain. They are involved in memory and in particular long term memory. There are some schools of thought who believe it is through better understanding of these receptors that there will be breakthroughs in medication for such illnesses as Alzheimer's.

http://www.mdpi.com/1422-0067/16/1/547

We also know from this same paper that – (-) linalool plays an active part in ATP-sensitive K+ channels.

Say what?

I know. It's like another language isn't it!!!

In short, these are the channels that open and close the gateways of insulin and control diabetes.

But...

I have come across K+ channels before in a book I started to write before and got entirely boxed in by a brand new piece of research about a genetic mutation called TRESK K+. Discovered in 2010, this is one of the biggest breakthroughs in understanding migraine, especially those who experience the visual disturbances that accompany it also known as "aura". Whilst it is has only been identified in one family of sufferers of familial hemiplegic migraine and never in any other sufferer so far (and thus none of us is likely to have it) it does give valuable insights to researchers trying to design treatments for migraine.

TRESK is a potassium ion channel. Its job is to help potassium to leave cells. The genes involved in moving salts around the body are more correctly known as ion channels or transporter genes. They can determine how easily our nerves become excited and they also dictate how they react to stimulus. The mutation that was discovered disrupted how efficiently the ion channel worked.

For many years migraine was thought to be either a disorder of blood vessels or perhaps a problem with inflammation. It is now, however, generally accepted that migraine should be considered a disorder of the nervous system. Studies show consistent findings that migraine sufferers experience an increased nervous responsiveness to stimulation, even between attacks. Since the degree to which a nerve channel can be excited is dependent on ion channels, anomalies in these genes might also explain why migraine sufferers' nervous systems are more excitable.

And Basil...our foremost essential oil for mental clarity and headaches....also affects these channels.

Lungs

Acute lung injuries were induced on mice in a lab in Jilin University, China in 2013. Linalool reduced the strength of signals that triggered interleukin 5 (remember the inflammation cytokines?) and also tumour necrosis-α leading to the conclusion statement of the study that linalool *"may be a potential therapeutic candidate for the treatment of inflammatory diseases."*

Emotions and Neurological responses

A Brazilian trial from 2009 examined the effects that Basil had on epileptic fits, and sought to understand exactly how Basil was doing its job. Our little Swiss mice are the stars of the show again and were injected with different types of drugs to induce fitting. Each drug, flumazenil,

Diazepam, Sodium thiopental, Pentylenetetrazol, Pictrotoxin had been chosen because of the scientist's understanding of how it worked on the body.

In some cases, the essential oil raised the hypnotic effect of the drug, in others it prevented convulsions. This demonstrated to them the linalool (which they identified as being the active component) was acting on the body through the GABA receptors.

A quick physiology recap for you: GABA receptors (Gamma Aminobutyric Acid) are neurotransmitters and some of the most important aspects of our chemical nervous system. They are responsible for excitability of the nervous system but they also regulate smooth muscle.

This gives us a tiny bit more into how Basil works as an antidepressant too. You'll remember that the same discoveries were found when they were working with investigations into rose too.

http://www.redalyc.org/pdf/856/85611774006.pdf

Antioxidant

A 2010 study from the Journal of Agricultural and Food Chemistry looked at the relative anti-oxidant properties of essential oils. Thyme fared the best in the all of the assays (scoring between 80-100%), but Basil scored a massive 86% success rate in scavenging the harmful free radicals that degrade our cells.

Pesto for dinner, I think, guys. Don't you?

However I think it is worth quoting a 2008 article from The Journal of Agricultural and Food Chemistry, which was interested in the fact that, whilst there are huge range of biological and pharmacological properties proven for Sweet Basil, this is still not yet dependable data. This is because the results indicate that in vitro anti-oxidant activity is not predictive of biological activity (that is to say just because it works in a test tube, we cannot guarantee the body will work in the same way) and also that Basil will offer different levels of protection based on its composition. So, again we have this throw back to Ethnobotany that says it is not just the species that makes the difference, but the soil and conditions it has grown in and thus its chemistry. Lastly, of course, with Basil more than most essential oils/plants, there are a vast array of cultivars all performing differently (just look at Holy Basil for example; it is starkly different in the way it acts). We can take these as indicators, prescriptors, nothing more. If we could...then the drugs company would have found a way to patent it by now. Their quest goes on and as therapists it is our job to watch, think and report. Your observations into how your Basil oil works is every bit as valid as that of Dioscorides or even the man with the goggles and the Bunsen burner...

Not least, because essential oils and Basil more than any other oil I know will execute magic differently on everyone who uses them. The end destination of happiness, confidence, better digestion et al, will be the same, but the map you read to get there will look very different for everyone I think.

Ear Ache

Scientists in Iceland wanted to investigate the effects of Basil versus a placebo (olive oil) against poorly rat ears. Now this is an interesting study because it is all done by vapour treatment. The tympanic membrane is not considered to be permeable to liquids but the researchers suspected that they might be able to get the vapours to diffuse from the external ear canal into the middle ear in large enough quantities for the antimicrobial molecules to do their work.

So they infected 113 rodents with pneumococci and 75 with Haemophilus influenzi on day one of the trial then started on their treatment on the second day after infection. 15 rats in each group were treated with Basil. Then the Basil treatment was compared with cocktails of essential oil *constituents*. A double mixture contained 4 g of thymol, 4 g of carvacrol and 92 g of ethanol (96% solution). The triple mixture contained 4 g of thymol, 4 g of carvacrol, 2 g of salicylaldehyde, and 90 g of ethanol (96% solution)

They placed a piece of cotton wool with two drops of oil into the ear (and plugged it with a little piece of plastic clay to hold it in place whilst the rat slept.) To exclude the possibility that a slightly different ear problem called *acute otitis externa* might play a role in curing acute otitis *media*, acute otitis externa was provoked by rotating a wooden pin against the external ear canal in 8 rats infected with pneumococci.

There was improvement in acute otitis media in the pneumococci rats after just 1 day of treatment (so that would be the third day after infection) with Basil oil Swabs were taken from their ears and discharge from 2 rats had improved from being *purulent* to being *mixed purulent and clear*.

After two days of treatment (fourth after infection), another 20 Basil rats had improved, whereas only four of the control rats were getting better. In addition to this, three Basil rats had clear swabs whereas only two control rats had.

Day 5 after infection, eight (53%) of fifteen Basil rats were cured, whereas only one (6%) of the control group was cured. Disappointingly though even after the third treatment with Basil, all rats had still developed acute otitis externa (and I can't find any trials yet that suggest they might have found answers for that).

http://jid.oxfordjournals.org/content/191/11/1876.full

Kidney

Those of you have diabetes, or diabetics in the family will know that for sufferers, the kidneys are of primary concern. This is because they become more prone to injury, oxidative stress and cell abnormalities. So, a team Annamalai University in India wanted to see what linalool might be able to do to help that, so they created some diabetic rats and then treated them with linalool for 45 days.

On appraisal it was found that the diabetic rats' glucose was being metabolised differently because the linalool had restored the metabolising enzymes. The kidney had been protected from oxidative stress and inflammation

http://informahealthcare.com/doi/abs/10.3109/15376516.2012.743638

Mouth

Forty patients were selected for a 21 day study comparing the effectiveness of herbal mouth washes versus commercial ones. Plaque and gingivitis were measured at baseline recruitment, after 14 days and 21 days. Sadly the trial does not discuss how it created the mouthwash, just that it contained tea tree, close and sweet Basil. It is a bit of a strange trial because it compares the results against an existing herbal mouth rinse with the same ingredients, so one can only draw the conclusion this is for a new patent perhaps. Anyhoo...

Results showed that gingivitis and plaque were both effectively reduced by both the existing and this new formulation.

http://www.ncbi.nlm.nih.gov/pubmed/25024544

Acne

In 2012 Universidad de Cartagena, Columbia declared that since acne strains of bacteria have developed anti-microbial resistance then alternatives to anti-biotic treatments have become necessary.

A very simple study was trialled using gel formulations versus a medication. The gels were comprised of

- Antibacterial essential oils. Orange oil was compared against the actions of Basil oil.

- Kerolytic medication

- Essential oils mixed with acetic acid

- Acetic acid and kerolytic medication.

28 volunteers separated into groups of seven patients. Treatments were applied daily for 8 weeks.

In case you are not familiar with acetic acid, it is the major component of vinegar, but in vinegar it is only a dilution of about 5% so that is a very weak example.

Actually all of the treatments fared well, with the kerolytic on its own being the least effective with a 43% improvement (which is still quite effective isn't it?). Orange saw a 51.4% improvement, Basil 60.95%

improvement, but the mixture of orange and Basil with the acetic acid was 75% improvement. It was thought that the stripping action of the acid pared with the keratolytic activity (growth of new skin cells) were the reasons for this although the authors did acknowledge that smelling like a fish and chip shop might be a significant downside here!

http://www.scielo.org.co/pdf/bio/v32n1/v32n1a14.pdf

Insect Repellent
For Chucks!

Again we are on linalool investigations here more than Basil, but it made me smile and I can imagine some of the small holders amongst you loving this one, especially my li'l sis, Angela.

This is an article from Poultry Science in 2014, where a team from Southern Plains Agricultural Research Centre in Texas were looking to seriously improve the lot of their chickens. They wanted to assess anti microbial and insect repellent properties so linalool was added to the diets of chicks on the day they hatched and were fed linalool supplemented diets for 3 weeks. They established that the properties were best achieved in a dilution of 2% or less (at

147

5% their livers became really heavy), to get rid of bugs, keep them healthy and also...and I loved this...calm.

I like this team!

http://www.ncbi.nlm.nih.gov/pubmed/24570447

E- Coli

Basil and Rosemary were trialled against 60 different strains of Escherichia Coli. The clinical trains were taken from the respiratory tracts of patients. . Both oils inhibited the growth of the bacteria, with Basil doing it better.

You should read this paper because it really puts the importance of our oils into perspective. All of the strains were resistant to the synthetic antibiotics and yet were inhibited by the oils.

"The results of our tests clearly demonstrate that Basil and rosemary essential oils can be widely used to eliminate clinical strains of Escherichia coli found in different clinical conditions."

The authors were also citing the following data that is useful to us:

*In our tests, Basil oil obtained from Ocimum Basilicum, containing **mainly estragole (86.4%)**, inhibited the growth all* strains isolated from various clinical materials. Among them were bacteria isolated from urine, which were also extended-spectrum beta-lactamase positive. Our studies confirm that antibacterial activity is possessed by not only Basil oil chemotypes with linalool or eugenol as their main components, but also that of Ocimum Basilicum, containing mainly estragole. Our research showed that **Basil essential oil was significantly more effective against all clinical isolates than rosemary essential oil.** Similar results were obtained by Hammer et al, who studied the antimicrobial activity of Basil and rosemary essential oils **against Acinetobacter baumanii, Aeromonas veronii biogroup sobria, Candida albicans, Enterococcus faecalis, Escherichia coli, Klebsiella pneumoniae, Pseudomonas aeruginosa, Salmonella enterica subsp. enterica serotype typhimurium, Serratia marcescens and Staphylococcus aureus,** using an agar dilution method. The authors confirmed that **Basil (Ocimum Basilicum) oil is more active against Escherichia coli than rosemary** (Rosmarinus officinalis). The MIC values were 0.5 and 1.0% (v/v), respectively. According to Lopez et al., the oils from Ocimum Basilicum and Rosmarinus officinalis have an **antibacterial potential against the Gram-positive bacteria Staphylococcus aureus, Enterococcus faecalis (Molecules 2013, 18 9345) and Listeria monocytogenes and against Gram-negative bacteria Escherichia coli, Yersinia**

149

enterocolitica, Salmonella choleraesuis and Pseudomonas aeruginosa as food borne bacterial strains. The authors present a detailed analysis of the tested oils and their ability to inhibit the growth of bacteria. Their Basil and rosemary essential oils were of a similar composition to the essential oils in our investigations

You can download the full paper at: http://www.mdpi.com/1420-3049/18/8/9334

Salmonella

A 2010 team from Ubon Ratchathani University in Thailand proved that Basil was effective in inhibiting the growth of bacteria injected into a pork sausage. The bacteria levels of salmonella were more than halved by the second day after treatment with Basil oil and were virtually undetectable by the third day. The study suggests that Basil oil might be of potential use as an antimicrobial agent to control Salmonella Enteritidis in food. The quantities, though, were tiny. They measured the oil in parts per million (ppm). The first day's reduction was achieved with 50ppm, and the eradication of the bacteria on the second day was at 100ppm, then on day 3 with 150ppm.

The problem they face now...and hence their further explorations...is that 150ppm would be too high to use at a general usage for population (although I don't see why, because it is below the FDA usage for food...perhaps it would taste too strong? Dunno...anyway, if you need to deal with any salmonella issues, Basil's your guy.!

http://www.ncbi.nlm.nih.gov/pubmed/20530897

Very quickly, apparently there are issues with histamines causing toxins in fresh fish when it is in storage, because of a bacterial species called Morganella morganii (amongst others). These toxins can cause severe allergic reactions, so clove, lemon grass and Basil were tested against them because they were seen as traditional Thai spices. Clove oil did the best job against them, followed by lemongrass and then our mate Basil.

http://www.ncbi.nlm.nih.gov/pubmed/23625419

Chapter 6 The Vibrational Medicine of Basil

Musical Note

Basil (linalool CT) vibrates on the musical note B flat. Whereas B flat minor is considered the chord of death because it is heard behind murder and suicide scenes in films, B flat major is bright cheerful, hopeful. Already that feels like a Basil conflict doesn't it?

I am blessed to havea condition called synesthesia that means I have two senses connected. Some musicians see colours in the tunes they play; I hear essential oils as musical notes. I hear Basil as a B Flat Major chord so you would have expected the songs to be hopeful. In fact, they are more aggressive and challenging, I would have said. Certainly there is no romance here. Don't expect to be floating off on tranquil sounds because that just is not Basil essence. Dancing and flirting though...oh yes there is plenty of that!

This part has been hard to write because, bizarrely, many of these songs were ones I played repeatedly in a very hard time of my life living with dangerously aggressive man. Some, I haven't heard for a long, long time and even I was shocked it was how cathartic it felt having a bottle of Basil in my hands as I played them. It felt like a wall separated me from the pain. Unusual, very odd and completely welcome! So here in the first songs we'll investigate the kind of emotions Basil helps. As we know she is not soft and floaty and so at the very beginning of her use, neither are the emotions you use her for. They are spiteful, angry, confused and conflicted. Remember your theme will be some kind of perception of the emotions being ready to explode (or implode!) in someone who is repressing them, or their having an icily cold demeanour because of them.

Prepare yourself. The first doors we are going to open are painful. For those of you with a gentle constitution....you'll want to turn the volume down!

To make it simple, I have added all the songs into one playlist for you here: http://tinyurl.com/oykzp54

(I know! Get me! Right?!) The downside is if you do have an addiction to bingo then you are going to spend a fortune with all the ads in between the songs and some seriously dodgy editing. I warned you there would be demons!

Basil oil for Pain

Crawling in my skin, these wounds they will not heal

Fear is how I feel, confusing what its real

Goddess, I remember this rage. The howling of anger, pain and fear that screamed inside my heart. *What should I do?* And yet every word that came out was careful and measured. There was a total disconnect between the physical me that people knew and the one yelling inside. That "me" was a necessary and deliberate creation, she went to work, achieved, in fact super achieved and she smiled. But when she went home...

I am not sure this song really requires much more explanation. If the smile on the face seems out of place, then I would always start with Basil.

Don't let the first couple of lines of this song defeat you. Chester Bennington's voice softens and becomes hauntingly enigmatic in this brilliant piece of music.

Crawling – Linkin Park

https://www.youtube.com/watch?v=6n6jN330vfU

Actually Linkin Park's Hybrid Theory album was given to me by my lovely husband, months after hell had frozen over and I had slammed the door permanently shut in this other man's face. I wonder what he saw in me that he felt it would be a good fit. I had not really even heard of the band, so it was a strange gift to give me but looking back now he must have sensed the fury...Listening now makes me wonder if it was seeping out of me- I don't know. But the next song resounds with me because it encapsulated the look in my parent eyes every time I went back to that man. Here, in this essay I can feel the Basil medicine for the narcissist's child who has impossible expectations to live up to and the fury that creates.

Numb –Linkin Park

https://www.youtube.com/watch?v=I2REZSj4XnE

It is odd listening to *Stan* **by** *Eminem* now because I can't remember being at all shocked by the intensity of it when it came out and I think that probably says a lot about the strange place my head was in.

The dichotomy of the narrative here appealed because we have poor Stanley becoming more and more consumed by obsession for his idol. He gets ever more aggressive and unbalanced and in the background we hear the bewildered wails of his heavily pregnant girlfriend. She is entirely in love with him, but he oblivious, his attention is dangerously elsewhere. She can see it is all getting out of hand, too hot, but telling him only lands her in a very scary place.

Since Basil energy is always un-tempered by thought and manners I felt that the uncensored version was the best link to post here.

Eminem- Stan

https://www.youtube.com/watch?v=IAPda9CigvY

This is how you remind me – Nickelback

I can remember dancing wildly to this every Friday and Saturday night, because it was safe. Then I bought the album and my kids would plead me to turn it off because they were sick to the back teeth of it. But this was the anthem of my torture.

These five words in my head

Scream "are we having fun yet?"

Yeah, yeah, yeah, *no, no*

Yeah, yeah, yeah, *no, no*

Some of the most descriptive words I have ever heard

I'm sick inside without a sense of feeling

Oh yeah, that is truly Basil medicine.

https://www.youtube.com/watch?v=ufbexgPyeJQ

And lastly in this much traumatised section, it seems only right that we should see the very beautiful Robert Downey Jr. and Elton John's tragic **I Want Love**.

Don't feel nothing, Just old Scars

Toughening up around my heart

So who is he? Tormentor or tormented? Not sure. Either. Both. Where did this pain start and end? It aches of self hatred and loathing doesn't it? Basil medicine.

I challenge you sing this song without hugging yourself into foetal position. It has got to be the most defensive song I have ever heard; simultaneously, it is beautiful and ugly in every beat. Song or actor, that does that, I wonder? What a genius combination.

https://www.youtube.com/watch?v=ufbexgPyeJQ

Basil's Sexy Energy

So what about the sexual angle to Basil, because there's certainly that, but it's not straightforward seduction though is it?

Well it's flirty, dangerous and rather full of itself if you don't mind my saying. And between you and me, I think that's goddamn irresistible! Ready to meet some naughty gals and some chaps who don't mind having a giggle at their own Basil vibration?

Well first let's start with our friend Lola Montez, just in case you haven't yet been introduced? I won't write much because we ripped the poor lass to pieces in the spiritual part. You'll be glad to meet my happier dimension of Basil, I am sure. Love her I do.

Lifting her skirt. Howling like a wolf...

You go girl!

Lola Montez - Volbeat

https://www.youtube.com/watch?v=7CspafvAui4

And what about **Michael Jackson's** *Dirty Diana?*

(And I'm not making any comments about Basil medicine and the artiste. You can work that one out for yourself. I'm just here for the dancing.)

Feel that pelvic chakra pulse of Basil and that fabulous whisper of B flat as it opens into fog.

https://www.youtube.com/watch?v=i-jgKhAB0k8

Then we've got animal prints out on patrol in *Sexy and I Know It*.

I love the line, "I've got passion in my pants and I'm not afraid to show it"

Who could resist that?

(Oops, sorry I drooled on the keyboard)

Do the wiggle dance!

Look at that body...

C'mon let's see you strut. Toss that head back. Jut that throat chakra out for everyone to see...express, baby !

https://www.youtube.com/watch?v=wyx6JDQCsIE&list=RDwyx6JDQCsIE

But we can't end this sex fest without my personal favourite Mars-gone-mad ballad **Kiss me I'm Sh**faced**

This poor fella should quit the beer and devour some pesto. I love his beer goggle honesty. If you haven't heard **The Dropkick Murphy's** delicious depiction of those guys in a bar who love themselves *way* too much, prepare yourself to giggle and flinch because it is very close to the bone. I will say this one is not for the faint hearted.

In the trousers she kissed me and I only bought her a round

It's so bad, it's funny. It's got to be said girls...I don't fancy yours much!

https://www.youtube.com/watch?v=7Aar_Mapjyw

Where Will Basil Take You?

Ok, so we understand who the medicine is for. But let's have a sense of what Basil can actually *do.* There are some good anthems here, I reckon. It is interesting how much dancing there are in the original videos of these and just as an side it strikes me that Basil does feel like that fantastic feeling of whipping fouetté pirouettes round and round; that delicious lightness of speed you feel in your head.

Let's start with **Elton John** drifting in space in **Rocket Man.** It's a dreamy start but there are a few thoughts in there I'd like you to consider. There are going to repercussions to your Basil outbursts and so I want you to prepare yourself for them. The chorus tells us the first thought:

And I think it's gonna be a long long time

Till touch down brings me round again to find

I'm not the man they think I am at home

Basil will change things. Know that. Don't use too much at once and make sure it is tempered by Venus ruled oils. Elton tells us why...

Mars ain't the kind of place to raise your kids

In fact it's cold as hell

Remember Basil is a short sharp shock...otherwise you are going to start being a person you really don't recognise as you. That's not fair on anyone. Baby steps please.

https://www.youtube.com/watch?v=-LX7WrHCaUA

Now let's visit the **Hall of Fame** and **The Script** with my belovéd **will.i.am**

You can throw your hands up

You can beat the clock (yeah)

You can move a mountain

You can break rocks

You can be a master

Don't wait for luck

Dedicate yourself and you gon' find yourself

The whole thing is Basil success but I love the idea that "you can walk through hell with a smile". Snook in there didn't it?

https://www.youtube.com/watch?v=mk48xRzuNvA

Mellowing right out now is the beautiful ballad by **John Mayer** called **Say**. It seems to address every aspect of being able to speak up when you need to. It is gentle, not forced and almost hymn-like in its simplicity. In the last lines, I can sense La Sirenne kneeling at the end of the bed with her sprig of Basil and whispering goodnight *Even as the eyes are closing* for the very last time.

Take all of your wasted honor

Every little past frustration

Take all of your so-called problems,

Better put 'em in quotations

Say what you need to say [8x]

Walking like a one man army

Fighting with the shadows in your head

Living out the same old moment

Knowing you'd be better off instead,

If you could only . . .

Say what you need to say [8x]

Have no fear for giving in

Have no fear for giving over

You'd better know that in the end

It's better to say too much

Than never to say what you need to say again

Even if your hands are shaking

And your faith is broken

Even as the eyes are closing

Do it with a heart wide open (a wide heart)

https://www.youtube.com/watch?v=7JONA_6ZCrE

We're nearly at the end now and I can't help but include the anthem of my publishing company Build Your Own Reality and my mission statement in every book I write. I love **Brave** by **Sarah Bareilles** and her thoughts that you can be the backlash of somebody's lack of love. (Ultimately scorpion, don't you think?)

You can be amazing

You can turn a phrase into a weapon or a drug

You can be the outcast

Or be the backlash of somebody's lack of love

Or you can start speaking up

Nothing's gonna hurt you the way that words do

When they settle 'neath your skin

Kept on the inside and no sunlight

Sometimes a shadow wins

But I wonder what would happen if you

Say what you wanna say

And let the words fall out

Honestly I wanna see you be brave

With what you want to say

And let the words fall out

Honestly I wanna see you be brave

https://www.youtube.com/watch?v=QUQsqBqxoR4

Given our delightful encounter with the dropkick Murphy's in the bar earlier, it's no surprise that **Sisters are Doing It for Themselves**. Ezulie Dantor wants to know what on Earth you need a man for anyway?! Remember our fantastic soldier lady rocking her beer on the dance floor?

Let's get up there and join her.

I want to see you standing on your own two feet. Ringing on your own bells

Sing it girls....

https://www.youtube.com/watch?v=drGx7JkFSp4

I'll leave the closing thoughts to the ever surprising **Sidewalk Prophets** and their prayerful song **The Words I Would Say**. Basil's protective energy connecting you to spirit, guiding you through fear to the wonderful success you can achieve. It's through tears that I sing to you

"I know 'cause I've already been there, so please hear these simple truths". No matter how desperate your situation feels, how dark it feels right now, trust in Basil and the universe's ability to shift and adjust to find you a way out. Focus your attention inwards and listen. You will find courage...from somewhere.

Be strong in the Lord and

never give up hope.

You're gonna do great things

I already know

God's got his hand on you so

don't live life in fear

forgive and forget

but don't forget why you're here

Take your time and pray

These are the words I would say

https://www.youtube.com/watch?v=8t9u-LOa3OI&list=RD8t9u-LOa3OI

Scorpion medicine, patience, strength, faith...Basil medicine.

Chapter 7 Basil Recipes

In this book more than any other, I think it becomes clear why, in many ways this recipe section is utter nonsense! The skill of the healer comes from determining the source of imbalance on a patient by patient basis. As ever this is designed as an assurance that you use your bottle of oil as much as you can – to get the most of the medicine. These are my thoughts, nothing more.

If this is the first of my books that you have read, let me explain that you will find no details of how to mix potions etc here. You will need to download my free book The Complete Guide to Clinical Aromatherapy and The Essential Oils of The Physical Body for that and you can find a direct link in the <u>"Other Books"</u> section at the back.

I found this blending research exciting and fascinating to do because I have followed the rule **to <u>temper Mars with Venus</u>** and then I have **<u>balanced the yang nature of Basil with an oil that has a yin softer element to it</u>**. Also recently Sedona Aromatherapy published a blog post about fruit carrier oils which encouraged me to experiment with some that I have never used before. Since red fruits fall under the planet of Venus, that has been exciting too, and the fragrance in the shed is pretty awesome today!

Lastly remember, this is my magic. It works because of my insights into patients I treat and people I know. Yours will be different. Think around the symptom and listen to the wisdom of your plants...then create your own recipes. That's when you will feel the magic crackle in your hands. (And don't think you need to go and buy all of these carrier oils...I am playing luxury experiments here, nothing more. Carrier oils do have their own properties and they will improve the benefits and the texture of products you make, but you certainly don't need as many as I have here! Check out Oshadhi's lists for an extensive number to play with.)

Key:

x 1 = 1 drop

x 2 = 2 drops etc

Cough

28ml (1oz) Peach Kernel Carrier Oil

Monarda x 2

Myrtle x 3

Basil x 1

Violet Leaf x 1

Rub three times daily over the throat.

Asthma

28ml (1oz) Almond Carrier Oil

Basil x 1

Frankincense x 4

Vetiver x1

Rub over the chest and back 3 times a day.

Chest Infection

28ml (1oz) Borage Carrier Oil

1 tsp Sea Buckthorn Carrier Oil

Basil x 1

Benzoin x 3

Cajuput x 1

Acne

I made a moisturiser here, but you could make a masque, toner, scrub... whatever you want. Just be aware of the delicate nature of acnied skin though, be gentle!

28ml (1oz) Blank Moisturiser

1 tsp Jasmine Maceration Oil

Basil x 1

Sweet Orange x 1

Jasmine absolute x 2

Tea tree x 1

Tummy Bug

28 ml (1 oz) Camomile maceration *(picked flowers from the garden then left them to steep in equal volume of sunflower oil for 28 days, then strained)*

1 x Basil

2 x cardamom

1 x mandarin

Massage over the abdomen, very lightly in a clockwise direction. Very lightly over the pelvis please.

Cold, Aching Joints

28ml (1oz) Tamanu Carrier Oil

Basil x 1

Black Pepper x 1

Geranium x 1

Scant Periods

100ml (4oz) Rosehip Carrier Oil

Basil x 4

Myrrh x 4

Rose x 4

Massage across the pelvis and lower back as often as you remember when you go to the toilet. Use for two cycles.

Fluid Retention

28ml (1oz) Red Raspberry Seed Carrier Oil

Basil x 1

Cypress x 3

Fennel x 1

I made this for menstrual massiveness, but you could use for puffy ankles just the same. Please don't use this in pregnancy though.

Headaches

28ml (1oz) Borage Carrier Oil

Basil x 1

Lavender x 1

Rosemary x 1

Angelica x 1

Massage onto the back of the neck, temples and pinch into the webbing between the thumb and first finger. Apply every 20 mins until the headache passes.

Emotional blends

I use these in a bowl of warm water or in the bath, but you can also use in a diffuser.

Open the windows

and let those "I am feeling like a victim" thoughts fly out

Basil x 1

Monarda x 1

Geranium x 1

Quit Being So Wet!

Hey, that's Basil speaking, I ain't saying nuffin!

Time to get the big girl pants on?

Watch it. This really is pants on fire medicine!

Basil x 2

Vetiver x 1

Black Pepper x 2

Private Pesto!

A little bit of Basil sauce for the bedroom ladies? (See what I did there?!)

I was excited to get my bottle of Tonka Bean out, because it is rarely sees the light of day, due to its (choking cough and splutter) price tag. But since Jill Bruce lists it as the oil of courtesans and seduction in *The Garden of Eden*, I thought we could choose it to channel our Inner Lola.

Don't ask if it works, I'll blush and so will my man! The bottle will be having more use from now on methinks! Just sayin'!

28ml (1oz) Rose Petal maceration Carrier Oil

Basil x 1

Tonka Bean x 1

Vetiver x 1

(It's too expensive to drop neat into the bath or evaporator so I made the mix and then drew from the mix)

Chapter 8 Conclusion

Well that was weird wasn't it? No-airy-fairy-isn't-aromatherapy-just-lovely- let's- just- float-on-a-cloud here, was there?! I found the whole journey entirely fascinating, but I am glad it is over! What I will say though is, boy, am I smiling a lot more!

In the music part I spoke of how Basil makes you feel like a fouetté pirouette. Pertinently fouetté means whipped...as in you whip them round and round. I do feel like that has happened to me this month. My world has been turned upside down with it and I genuinely feel dizzy with it. Just in case you don't have a point of reference for this (**http://tinyurl.com/oz4ygd2** - Mariella Nunez...not me!)

Many very important doors have opened to me this month, and I only had to knock with the very lightest of taps. Not least this lovely new association with Oshadhi. Please do pop over to them and look them up. Their oils are exquisite, but there is a bigger ethical picture at play here too. With the massive upsurge in interest in aromatherapy, and more specifically essential oils, massive pressure is being put on the world's oils resources. Usage of oils such as agarwood, sandalwood and rosewood mean that they are now in limited supply

176

as are the trees and forests they are being taken from, sadly. Promotion on oils such as Blue Tansy have meant that, not only is it harder to obtain, but adulteration has become very widespread. We need artisan distillers to keep aromatherapy "cleaner" but also to give some of the overly intensified areas of farming a well deserved break. Often these smaller distillers depend on trade from the likes of you and me to keep an entire village in work and food. Here you can make a very real difference, and in return you receive a superior product. By all means carry on shopping at "the big two" and other larger producers but know that you are getting the Tesco equivalent to an exclusive delicatessen.

In short...you get what you pay for.

I thought you might like to see something else I have been working on involving Basil.

She appears with the words "Basil is bossy" when a new friend of mine, Bertie the Bumblebee, accidentally falls headlong into my herb garden and the adventures he has learning about medicinal plant. My illustrator, Robert Elsmore, is bringing my poem to life with some adorable pictures.

This is an early line drawing of Bertie looking very morose (because he feels poorly) under lavender as he first meets his new friend Dexter the Dragonfly. These two get into all sorts of a pickle with Isla the Wide Eyed Frog

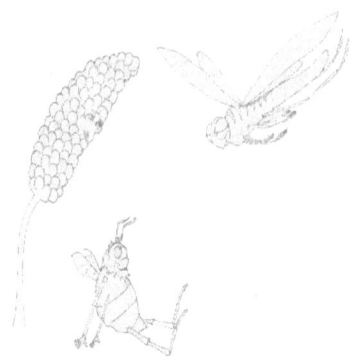

before being saved by some rather special herbs....

This colour- illustrated children's book should, I hope, go in sale Sept 2015.

I'd like to thank all of you who have done your never ending promoting for me. It has opened doors for me that I might only have been able to dream of otherwise. It is too early to give away too much information, but it seems likely that I might be able to offer training solutions for some of you who want to become qualified aromatherapists from next year.

Thank you for all your email and lovely messages. Your questions have kept me on my toes this month and I have learned a lot of new things. I would like to give a wave to a lady who emails me to say, just hi, every month without fail. Her name is Zuzana Garajova. Also to Connie Valenti who single-handedly doubled the total sales of my Monarda book in one afternoon, just by shouting up for me when someone posted a picture of the plant. Actions like that make a massive difference to me and make it possible for me to be able to afford to give books away on their launch date. The next oils book – Melissa - is dedicated to them. Thanks both of you, you are very much appreciated.

I opened this book with a dedication to Lynda Jaffray, who plummeted into the depths of despair after being profoundly affected by a traumatic event...and found she was a different person entirely. Lynda turns up on Facebook so often and always has something wonderful to say. She sends me source material and contacts and even stories of mystical books. She is one of the few people I have ever encountered who smiles at ancient philosophies almost as much as I do. It is lovely to have found such a kindred spirit.

You can always find her easily because there will be a massive kissing unicorn or similar emoticon next to her details. I know her well through her posts and always have an inkling which ones will spark her, but I realised I knew nothing about her life at all. When I asked her she wrote:

I'm 58 years old and could fill a book with my life story which I hope to do one day. I got married at 16 and have been married for 42 years to my darling husband who was in the Army for 32 years and we travelled some of the world together along with our children. I have two children and two grandchildren and adore being a Granny. I was drawn to holistic healing about 5 years ago when a traumatic event occurred in my life and I plummeted into the depths of despair which was a major turning point in my life and in my belief system. I went on to train in several complementary therapies and qualified to practitioner level in Indian Head massage, Reflexology, Aromatherapy and 1st & 2nd degree Reiki and along the way met some amazing women. I do not have my own practice as yet but have the intention of setting up my own business in the not too distant future. I feel I still have lots to learn and I am enjoying the journey and look forward to the day that I can help others to heal.

I have chosen not to ask her about the trauma, given the nature of the book I have written in her name but I am heartened to know that her life is renewed. Lynda is a very treasured lady and I am very grateful for all her support and friendship.

One last (more than a little creepy) thing I will share with you before I go. I have been treating a patient with a hideous cough. She has had this affliction for three years now and the doctors are perplexed. I have been using Basil in a cream I gave her and I checked in a couple of days after first giving it to her. She sent me a text saying she felt she was coughing less but had decided to take some time off work. She said "I am sure you have guessed I am a bit of a hoarder" (I hadn't at all) "I have been cleaning and tidying, throwing things out, which isn't like me at all!"

I looked around me. So had I! And I mean really tidying on a supercharged scale...which really isn't like me either! I emptied boxes in the bedroom that had been there since we moved into the cottage three years ago. I had even put flowers and pot pourri in the bedroom, which has been a dumping ground since we moved in. The office in the shed has turned into a sanctuary for cardboard butterflies and it looks distinctly girly!

Could it be I saw a flash of a beautiful blonde lady with dancing green eyes? She seemed to look up and smirk at me as she filed her nails...Ezulie Freda? Did you do this? Thanks if you did, because it felt ace and after grimacing at the mess for months, it was effortless! Dunno...seriously weird though!

The scope of Basil is too big to sum up, isn't it? I dare you to try and explain the Mars- Linalol – Scorpio journey to someone who tells you to put a couple of drops of Basil in your glass of water each day! That'll shut them up for a moment at least.

So I am going to finish by heading back one last time to the songs and say

Grab your bottle of Basil and make some changes.

Show me...

How big your brave is!

Lots of love

Liz

PS Don't forget to review and buy!

Bye xxx

PPS If you would like to join my mailing list pop over to facebook.com/TheSecretHealerWrites and click the email list link.

Other books in The Secret Healer Series

Available in ebook and paperback formats.

The Essential Oils Profiles

<u>Monarda – A Native American Medicine</u>

<u>Vetiver – An Ayurvedic Medicine</u>

<u>Holy Basil – An Ayurvedic Medicine</u>

<u>Rose – Goddess Medicine</u> (also available as an illustrated paperback)

Coming soon....

Melissa

Patchouli

And the first of Bertie Bumble's adventures in The Secret Healer's Garden.

To get the very best from your learning experience, why not treat yourself to one of the Secret Healer Training Manuals? To begin with, have you taken advantage of the free essential oil profiles available in...?

Book 1 - The Complete Guide to

Clinical Aromatherapy & Essential Oils for the Physical Body

Essentially...essential oils for beginners, talented novices and intermediate aromatherapists

Let me ask you, why do you want a book on aromatherapy?

Do you want to learn how to care for your family naturally?

Perhaps you have a franchise selling essential oils and want to know more about what they can do?

Maybe you love the delicious scents and want understand how these beautiful things come to heal.

I wonder if you have started to learn and now want to discover how to build on your knowledge.

Whatever you are looking for this book has something for you.

Details of how to treat over 60 conditions with essential oils

Profiles of over 100 natural plant essences and their safety data

Descriptions of 15 carrier oils and their applications not only for massage but also adding to creams and lotions.

Comprehensive data of how the chemistry of an oil will affect its actions

In depth insights into how professional aromatherapists blend...including their 13 favourite recipes from their practices.

Including....

Sensuous aromatherapy blends by a qualified sex therapist

Two blends for labour by the midwife running an aromatherapy program on an NHS maternity ward

A blend for depression by a qualified mental health

PLUS....

10 bonus essential oil monographs and a complementary hypnotherapy relaxation download.

Discount vouchers of treatments courses and products by participating therapists.

AND.... for those of you who would like to contribute, there is a chance to make a donation to cancer research too.

This is my gift to you.

Download for FREE -

Book 2 Essential Oils for Mind Body Spirit

The Holistic Medicine of Clinical Aromatherapy

Healing the skin, easing the tummy ache or getting someone to sleep is easy with essential oils. Anyone can do it. The joy of healing, though, comes from peeling back the layers of the disease, almost like a detective to find out exactly what caused it in the first place.

Consider this book to be lesson 2 in The Secret Healer Series.

You have mastered which oil to use for what and why...this book takes you step by step though the ancient healing mechanisms of the aura, the chakras and meridians but also explores how that ties in with the latest scientific discoveries into how the emotions affect our health. Using Candace Pert's remarkable "Molecules of

Emotion" research, The Secret Healer shows you *where* to look for healing links and *why*.

Uncover how a certain recurrent negative emotion can be the trigger to make you ill?

Understand internal processes that mean that psychology, neurology and immunology are quintessentially, and inextricably linked.

Learn how to use essential oils control your emotions and in turn bring about a far greater standard of wellness.

Discover mind blowing research that shows the emotions we experience are actually the sensations of neuropeptides triggering our organs to do their jobs

Reflect on the wonder of Chinese medicine and ancient healing being completely accurate in their healing mechanisms for thousands of years...now that science proves it to be so.

Essential Oils for The Mind Body Spirit couples ancient wisdom with cutting edge science. This is the knowledge the drug companies hope you never find out and our doctors pray we all will.

A short write up, for a book that will change your life. I promise you, when you read the latest findings of psychoimmunolgy, you will never waster another day on being angry again.

Book 3 The Essential Oil Liver Cleanse

The Professional Aromatherapist's Liver Detox

We are warned of the threats of heart attacks, strokes and cancer, especially if we are overweight.

What is kept quieter is doctors have established a link between toxicity in the liver and metabolic syndrome, the condition that leads to many of these conditions. What's more non fatty liver disease is known to underlie many other conditions such as eczema, allergies and headaches.

The scandal is just how many of our livers are struggling under the strain of over processed foods, pharmaceutical debris and actually even our own bad tempers!

This book explains:

The importance of the liver and its functions

How it becomes dysfunctional and how to interpret warning signposts

How to cleanse and nourish using not just essential oils, but also vitamins and minerals and diet.

The strange correlation between how our emotions translate negativity into disease.

How to implement other therapies such as chiropractic, acupressure and counselling and how to secure fantastic referrals.

This book is best used in tandem with The Professional Stress Solution to benefit from the complementary healing. Use Sales Strategies for Gentle Souls to create a marketing plan to use your new found knowledge to smash your competition out of the water!!!

Book 4 The Professional Stress Solution

Essential Oils and Holistic Health Stress Management Techniques for The Professional Aromatherapist

Stress is pandemic in our society.

Scientists agree it plays a quintessential role in how likely it is we will suffer from chronic and possibly fatal illnesses in the future. Risk factors of metabolic syndrome, diabetes, stroke and heart disease are increased through stress.

The daft thing is....aromatherapy can do amazing things to ease it, and potentially aromatherapists could take a massive workload away from the doctor's surgeries.

Discover the hormonal changes and peptide triggers that change a person's health and mental state.

Learn how it affects the liver, adrenals and pituitary gland.

Uncover the strange phenomenon of Yin disease

Build a better foundation of care, but also a knowledge base that means you can sell your treatments more effectively.

Improve your healing skills set

Supercharge your referrals potential from other complementary therapists and orthodox medicine alike.

Includes free bonus material of

Chiropractic chart of misalignments and potential organic disturbance

Chart of the meridians and suggested acupressure points to detox the organs more quickly

Detailed information about how to improve the patients condition with vitamin and minerals therapy

In depth dietary advice

Free hypnotherapy relaxation download

Essential Oils are The Off Switch for stress. The *Professional Stress Solution* is the ON SWITCH for your aromatherapy business.

Book 5 The Aromatherapy Eczema Treatment

Healing Eczema, Itchy Skin Rashes and Atopic Dermatitis with Essential Oils and Holistic Medicine

Most people appreciate that the itching and redness of eczema can be used using essential oils, but what if I told you they were capable of so much more?

Imagine if, as a therapist, you were able to pinpoint the emotions that set off these flares? Can you visualise what it would mean to your patient if you were able to isolate the very protagonist causing the eczema breakout and alleviate their pain completely?

Well now you can.

This book teaches you:

How to isolate the emotions causing the emotional cycle of pain

The likely food triggers for your patient and the tools to identify the exact times they will detonate a reaction

The familial traits and links that lead to atopic eczema

How these links connect with the liver and in turn how to cleanse the liver toxicity

Vitamins and minerals to cleanse and nourish the system

The book contains very real that will not only transform the way you treat clients, but will skyrocket your clinic's takings.

I recommend reading this book in tandem with *The Professional Stress Solution* and the *Essential Oil Liver Cleanse* to fully understand the cycles and processes of treatment. Add to it *Sales Strategies for Gentle Souls* and your business will stand on an entirely new footing.

Sales Strategies for Gentle Souls

Targeted Sales Training for Professional Aromatherapists

Wonderful things are happening in complementary therapy. Very gifted people are churning out fantastic research and results. The internet is full of what essential oils can do. But when a gentle soul emerges from their relaxing haze of their aromatherapy class room, how do they harness the buzz of energy around them for their craft?

From 1999-2008 I worked in one of the most aggressive commercial environments there is. My role as a recruitment consultant was 80% cold calling in am extremely saturated sales arena. Despite my own gentle soul, I found ways not only to compete, but to excel.

Learn how to pinpoint the best customers for your practice

Cost your treatments to ensure every treatment is profitable for both you and your customer

Discover how to make every conversation into a potential sale lead without becoming a complete and utter pain in the a*s!

Uncover the reasons why you are not closing sales so you never have to make the same mistakes again

Create a growth environment where you plan success and always find yourself stepping into it

If you are working with essential oils, and you want to make a good living for it, then you need to learn to sell. What's more, if you are going to say "selling doesn't work on my customers"....then you have simply been taught to do it wrongly.

My dream is to see aromatherapy at the forefront of medicine. I need an army of gifted healers to achieve that. Consider yourself to be my newest recruit and I am going to drill you till you are the slickest, subtlest and most effective marketeer there is. You have the knowledge to make people better, now let me give you the business prowess to heal even more people than you have ever done before.

The Secret Healer has stress in her sights and she's about to make a killing. Listen carefully...she has much to tell you.

www.thesecrethealer.co.uk

www.buildyourownreality.com

About the Author

Elizabeth Ashley qualified as an aromatherapist in 1993, and then passed her Advanced Aromatherapy Diploma in 1994. She has been practicing aromatherapy for almost 22 years.

In 1999, she fell into a whole new career in the aggressive commercial sector of recruitment consultancy. There she discovered her father's second hand car salesman genes had passed along and found she had quite a gift of the gab! More than that, she discovered she could sell...and then some.

In 2008, Elizabeth fell ill during pregnancy with a blood clot in her lungs. The pulmonary embolism prevented her from working and she started to write. Very quickly she gained her first contract as a ghost writer...a recipe book for cheese cakes!

In 2010 she was published professionally for her work on Galbanum oil in the Aromatherapy Thymes, journal of the International Federation of Aromatherapists, and on Tuberose oil by the New Zealand Register of Holistic Therapist.

In 2011 she was seconded on a consultative basis to Walsall Independent Treatment Centre, designed to be a rainbow bridge between traditional and complementary medicines. There she became aware of the rumblings of change in healthcare. Her book *Sales Strategies for Gentle Souls* explains the connotations of this.

Many of her books are aimed at helping qualified aromatherapists to expand their healing repertoire and build their businesses. She also writes for people who have an interest in essential oils and want to learn how to heal. Her in depth essential oil profiles chart the healing properties of plants from the most arcane depths of historic folklore up to the scientific lab trials of today.

In 2014 she ranks in the top 50 contract writers on the freelancer marketplace Elance.com. She is the ghost writer of seven number one Amazon best sellers in the natural healing category. She lives in Shropshire with her husband and youngest son, kept company by their cat, the budgie and many shoals of tropical fish! Her elder son and daughter attend University and make her prouder than anything ever could.

Elizabeth Ashley is possibly one of the most published aromatherapy writers you have never heard of! By 2015, all of that will have changed. Elizabeth Ashley is *The Secret Healer*.

Bibliography

1. *About Vibrational Healing.* (2015). Retrieved 25 24, 2015, from Rose of Raphael.com: http://www.roseofraphael.com.au/pages/vibratio nal-healing

2. Alchemy Works. (2015). *Basil Ocimum Basilicum.* Retrieved 07 2015, 2015, from Alchemy Works: http://www.alchemy-works.com/ocimum_Basilicum.html

3. Andrews, S. A. (2013, 05 01). *Basking In the Glory Of Basil.* Retrieved 07 20, 2015, from Humane Living: http://humanelivingnet.net/2013/05/01/basking-in-the-glory-of-Basil/

4. Archai. (2011). *The Planets.* Retrieved 07 20, 2015, from Archai The Journal of Archetypal Cosmology: http://www.archaijournal.org/planets.html#mars

5. Bartow, b. J. (Unlisted). *Scorpio.* Retrieved 07 20, 2015, from Living Spirit: http://www.livingspiritcommunity.net/Education /Archives/FollowtheSun/Sign-Archetypes/Scorpio.html

6. *Basil.* (2002). Retrieved 07 2015, 2015, from Iranica Online:

http://www.iranicaonline.org/articles/Basil

7. *Basilisk.* (2009). Retrieved 07 20, 2015, from Monstrous.com:

http://monsters.monstrous.com/Basilisk.htm

8. Beier RC1, B. J. (2013, 02). *Evaluation of linalool, a natural antimicrobial and insecticidal essential oil from Basil: effects on poultry.* Retrieved 07 20, 2015, from Pubmed:

http://www.ncbi.nlm.nih.gov/pubmed/24570447

9. Benardis, M. (2013). *Cooking & Eating Wisdom for Better Health: How the Wisdom of Ancient Greece Can Lead to a Longer Life.* Balboa Press.

10. Bruce, J. (1994). *The Garden of Eden .* Magdelena Press.

11. Cunningham, S. (2009). *Cunningham's Encyclopoedia of Magical Herbs.* Llewelyns.

12. *Cyclodextrin-Complexed Ocimum Basilicum Leaves Essential Oil Increases Fos Protein Expression in the Central Nervous System and Produce an Antihyperalgesic Effect in Animal Models for*

Fibromyalgia. (2014, 09 14). Retrieved 07 20, 2015, from Intyernational Journal of Molecular Sciences: http://www.mdpi.com/1422-0067/16/1/547

13. D'Andrea, J. *Ancient Herbs in the J. Paul Getty Museum Gardens.* Getty Publications; Reprint edition (Feb. 1983).

14. Dash, M. (2013, 07 23). *On The Trail Of The Warsaw Basilisk.* Retrieved 07 20, 2015, from Smithsonian: http://www.smithsonianmag.com/history/on-the-trail-of-the-warsaw-Basilisk-5691840/?no-ist

15. Davis, P. (2005). *Aromatherapy An A-Z: The most comprehensive guide to aromatherapy ever published.* Vermilion; Rev Ed edition.

16. DeVries, L. (2015). *Basil.* Retrieved 07 20, 2015, from Medicinal Herb Info: http://medicinalherbinfo.org/herbs/Basil.html

17. *Erzule Voodoo Goddessof Love.* (2015). Retrieved 07 20, 2015, from Love of The Goddess: http://loveofthegoddess.blogspot.co.uk/2013/05/erzulie-voodoo-goddess-of-love.html

18. *Erzulie*. (2013). Retrieved 07 20, 2015, from A-muse-ing Grace Gallery: http://www.thaliatook.com/AMGG/erzulie.php

19. *Erzullie Dantor*. (2010). Retrieved 07 20, 2015, from L Belle Deesse: http://www.labelledeesse.com/erzuliedantor.html

20. *Ezulie Freda Veve Sign* . (2011, 10 20). Retrieved 07 20, 2015, from Perkerburghs Hauntings: http://parkersburgghosts.blogspot.co.uk/2011/10/erzulie-freda-veve-sign.html

21. Gade Nou Leve Society. (Unlisted). *Ezili Danto*. Retrieved 07 20, 2015, from Gade Nou Leve : http://www.ezilikonnen.com/the-lwa/ezili-danto/

22. Gainsburgh, A. (2015). *The Journey of Mars The Drive of Desire*. Retrieved 07 20, 2015, from Soul Sign: http://www.soulsign.com/articles/the-journey-of-mars-the-drive-of-desire

23. Germán Matiz1, M. R. (2011, 08 23). *Diseño y evaluación in vivo de fórmulas para acné basadas en aceites esenciales de naranja (Citrus sinensis), albahaca (Ocimum Basilicum L) y ácido acético*. Retrieved 07 20,

2015, from Biomedica: http://www.scielo.org.co/scielo.php?script=sci_art text&pid=S0120-41572012000100014&lng=en&nrm=iso&tlng=en

24. Green, J. W. (2010, 10 17). Scorpio *Archetype*. Retrieved 07 20, 2015, from School of Evolutionary Aromatherapy: http://schoolofevolutionaryastrology.com/forum/index.php/topic,334.0.html

25. Hardy, J. (2014). *http://www.ediciones-narayana.es/homoeopathie/pdf/Spider-and-Scorpion-Remedies-in-Homeopathy-.15912.pdf.* Retrieved 07 20, 2015, from Narayana Verlag: http://www.ediciones-narayana.es/homoeopathie/pdf/Spider-and-Scorpion-Remedies-in-Homeopathy-.15912.pdf

26. Hermesh, C. (2012). *Scorpion.* Retrieved 07 20, 2015, from Spirit Animal Totems : http://www.spirit-animals.com/scorpion/

27. Holt, L. (2012, 12 02). *Basil Herbal Lore and Legends.* Retrieved 07 20, 2015, from Mother Earth Living: http://www.motherearthliving.com/natural-health/Basil-herbal-lore-and-legends.aspx

28. John M. Grohol, P. (2012). *Differences Between a Psychopath vs Sociopath*. Retrieved 07 20, 2015, from PsychCentral: http://psychcentral.com/blog/archives/2015/02/12/differences-between-a-psychopath-vs-sociopath/

29. Juliana S OLIVEIRAa, 1. L. (2009). *Phytochemical screening and anticonvulsant property of Ocimum Basilicum leafessential oil*. Retrieved 07 20, 2015, from http://www.redalyc.org/pdf/856/85611774006.pdf

30. Kathy. (2012, 11 12). *The Story of Ocimum Basilicum: Malevolent Beast or Ally and Protector?* Retrieved 07 20, 2015, from Redroot Mountain School of Botanical Medicine: http://www.redrootmountain.com/the-story-of-ocimum-Basilicum-malevolent-beast-or-ally-and-protector/620

31. Kothiwale SV1, P. V. (2014, 05 18). *A comparative study of antiplaque and antigingivitis effects of herbal mouthrinse containing tea tree oil, clove, and Basil with commercially available essential oil mouthrinse.*

Retrieved 07 20, 2015, from Pubmed: http://www.ncbi.nlm.nih.gov/pubmed/25024544

32. Lawless, J. (1992). *The Encyclopaedia of Essential Oils.* Dorset: Element Books .

33. Manniche, L. (1989). *An Egyptian Herbal* . London: British Museum Press.

34. Marceau, G. P. (2012). *The Sacred Masculine The12 Archetypes of Mars.* Retrieved 07 20, 2015, from Slideshare.net: http://www.slideshare.net/greggarceau/the-sacred-masculine-12-archetypes-of-mars

35. Medicinal Plants. (2011). *Basil: Contrary Opinions In The Tradition.* Retrieved 07 2015, 2015, from Medicinal Plants: http://medicinalplants.us/Basil-contrary-opinions-in-the-tradition

36. Meri, J. W. *Medieval Islamic Civilization: An Encyclopedia.* Routledge, 31 Oct 2005 .

37. Mojay, G. (1996). *Aromatherapy for Healing the Spirit: Restoring Emotional and Mental Balance with Essential Oils.* Tankabon.

38. Monika Sienkiewicz 1, *. ,. (2013). *The Potential of Use Basil and Rosemary Essential Oils as Effective Antibacterial Agents.* Retrieved 07 15, 2015, from Moelecules: http://www.mdpi.com/1420-3049/18/8/9334

39. Nelson, J. S. (2011, 08 07). *Plant Palate - Basil.* Retrieved 07 20, 2015, from University of Illinois: http://web.extension.illinois.edu/dmp/palette/110807.html

40. Nutripanda. (2014). *Basil both Salutary & Harmful .* Retrieved 07 20, 2015, from Nutripanda: http://www.nutripanda.com/Basil.html

41. O'Brien, P. (Unlisted). *Basil in TCM .* Retrieved 07 20, 2015, from How Foods Heal: http://www.meridian-acupuncture-clinic.com/support-files/Basil-in-tcm.pdf

42. *Ocimum Basilicum.* (Unlisted). Retrieved 07 20, 2015, from Ayushveda: http://www.ayushveda.com/herbs/ocimum-Basilicum.htm

43. OurHerb Garden . (2015). Retrieved 07 20, 2015, from Our Herb Garden :

http://www.ourherbgarden.com/herb-history/Basil.html

44. Patrick Lima, J. S. (2011). *The Organic Home Garden.* Five Rivers Chapmanry.

45. Rattanachaikunsopon P1, P. P. (2010). *Antimicrobial activity of Basil (Ocimum Basilicum) oil against Salmonella enteritidis in vitro and in food.* Retrieved 07 20, 2015, from PubMed: http://www.ncbi.nlm.nih.gov/pubmed/20530897

46. Reid, L. (Unlisted). *Archetypal Mars.* Retrieved 07 20, 2015, from sky script.co.uk: http://www.skyscript.co.uk/marsreid.html

47. Rich, V. A. *Cursing the Basil: And Other Folklore of the Garden.* Heritage House Pub Co Ltd, 2000.

48. Robin S. Edelstein, I. S. (2010, 08 01). *Narcissism Predicts Heightened Cortisol Reactivity to a Psychosocial Stressor in Men.* Retrieved 07 20, 2015, from Pubmed: http://www.ncbi.nlm.nih.gov/pmc/articles/PMC2976540/

49. Robin S. Edelstein, I. S. (2010, 10). *Narcissism Predicts Heightened Cortisol Reactivity to a Psychosocial*

Stressor in Men. Retrieved 07 20, 2015, from Pubmed: http://www.ncbi.nlm.nih.gov/pmc/articles/PMC2976540/

50. *Scorpion.* (2006). Retrieved 07 20, 2015, from Lins Domain: http://www.linsdomain.com/totems/pages/scorpion.htm

51. *Scorpion Medicine.* (04, 05 12). Retrieved 07 20, 2015, from Spirit Lodge: http://spiritlodge.yuku.com/topic/1006#.VazU5flViko

52. *Scorpion Stings: What To Use?* (2007, 02 15). Retrieved 07 20, 2015, from Homeopathy: http://www.homeopathyhome.com/forums/forum/homeopathy/homeopathy-list-discussion/8748-scorpion-stings-what-to-use

53. Sosyete du Marche Inc. (2015). *Ezulie Feda The Goddess of Love and Desire.* Retrieved 07 20, 2015, from Sosyete du Marche Inc: http://www.sosyetedumarche.com/html/erzulie_freda.html

54. Stenudd, S. (2015). Scorpio *Archetype*. Retrieved 07 20, 2015, from Scorpio Zodiac Sign: http://www.scorpiozodiacsign.net/scorpio-archetype.htm

55. That's Greece. (2015). *Basil The King Of The Herbs*. Retrieved 07 20, 2015, from That's Greece: http://www.thatsgreece.com/info/greek-cuisine-food-herbs-spices-Basil

56. *The Calling of Ezulie*. (Unlisted). Retrieved 07 20, 2015, from Comcast.net: https://home.comcast.net/~max555/rites/erzulie.html

57. The Herb Society Of America. (2003). *Basil*. Retrieved 07 20, 2015, from http://www.herbsociety.org/factsheets/Basil%20Guide.pdf

58. Tisserand, R. (1988). *Aromatherapy for Everyone*. London: Penguin Books.

59. Tisserand, R. (1977). *The Art of Aromatherapy*. Saffron Walden : The C. W Daniel Company Limited.

60. Venefica, A. (2015). *Symbol Meaning of Scorpion.* Retrieved 07 20, 2015, from Whats your sign.com: http://www.whats-your-sign.com/symbol-meaning-of-scorpion.html

61. West Texas Regional Poison Centre. (Unlisted). *Scorpions.* Retrieved 07 20, 2015, from Poison Centre: http://www.poisoncenter.org/poisonous-critters-1/scorpions

62. *What percentage of people are psychopaths / sociopaths?* (2011, 12). Retrieved 07 20, 2015, from Quora.com: https://www.quora.com/What-percentage-of-people-are-psychopaths-sociopaths

63. Wikipedia. (2015). *Erzulie.* Retrieved 07 20, 2015, from Wikipedia: https://en.wikipedia.org/wiki/Erzulie

64. Wildwood, C. (1996). *The Encyclopoeadia of Aromatherapy.* London: BloomsburyPublishing.

65. Woman, S. W. (2008, 04 19). *The Goddess Erzulie.* Retrieved 07 20, 2015, from Coven of The Goddess: http://www.covenofthegoddess.com/goddesserzulie.htm

66. Wood, M. (2008). *The Earthwise Herbal: A Complete Guide to Old World Medicinal Plants.* North Atlantic Books,U.S.

67. YourTango.com, C. H. (2013, 05 13). *Sociopath Signs: Is Your Ex A Sociopath Or A Narcissist?* Retrieved 07 20, 2015, from Huffington Post: http://www.huffingtonpost.com/2013/05/13/sociopath-signs-is-your-e_n_3181512.html

Disclaimer

by SEQ Legal

(1)   Introduction

This disclaimer governs the use of this ebook. [By using this ebook, you accept this disclaimer in full. / We will ask you to agree to this disclaimer before you can access the ebook.]

(2)   Credit

This disclaimer was created using an <u>SEQ Legal</u> template.

(3)   No advice

The ebook contains information about aromatherapy and the use of essential oils.The information is not advice, and should not be treated as such.

[You must not rely on the information in the ebook as an alternative to qualified medical advice from a health professional. advice from an appropriately qualified professional. If you have any specific questions about any medical matter you should consult an appropriately qualified professional.]

[If you think you may be suffering from any medical condition you should seek immediate medical attention. You should never delay seeking medical advice, disregard medical advice, or discontinue medical treatment because of information in the ebook.]

(4)   No representations or warranties

To the maximum extent permitted by applicable law and subject to section 6 below, we exclude all representations, warranties, undertakings and guarantees relating to the ebook.

Without prejudice to the generality of the foregoing paragraph, we do not represent, warrant, undertake or guarantee:

that the information in the ebook is correct, accurate, complete or non-misleading;

that the use of the guidance in the ebook will lead to any particular outcome or result; or

in particular, that by using the guidance in the ebook you will heal disease or work in any way as a cure for illness.

(5)   Limitations and exclusions of liability

The limitations and exclusions of liability set out in this section and elsewhere in this disclaimer: are subject to section 6 below; and govern all liabilities arising under the disclaimer or in relation to the ebook, including liabilities arising in contract, in tort (including negligence) and for breach of statutory duty.

We will not be liable to you in respect of any losses arising out of any event or events beyond our reasonable control.

We will not be liable to you in respect of any business losses, including without limitation loss of or damage to profits, income, revenue, use, production, anticipated savings, business, contracts, commercial opportunities or goodwill.

We will not be liable to you in respect of any loss or corruption of any data, database or software.

We will not be liable to you in respect of any special, indirect or consequential loss or damage.

(6) Exceptions

Nothing in this disclaimer shall: limit or exclude our liability for death or personal injury resulting from negligence; limit or exclude our liability for fraud or fraudulent misrepresentation; limit any of our liabilities in any way that is not permitted under applicable law; or exclude any of our liabilities that may not be excluded under applicable law.

(7) Severability

If a section of this disclaimer is determined by any court or other competent authority to be unlawful and/or unenforceable, the other sections of this disclaimer continue in effect.

If any unlawful and/or unenforceable section would be lawful or enforceable if part of it were deleted, that part will be deemed to be deleted, and the rest of the section will continue in effect.

(8)   Law and jurisdiction

This disclaimer will be governed by and construed in accordance with English law, and any disputes relating to this disclaimer will be subject to the exclusive jurisdiction of the courts of England and Wales.

(9)   Our details

In this disclaimer, "we" means (and "us" and "our" refer to) [individual name(s)] of [address(es)].

OR

In this disclaimer, "we" means (and "us" and "our" refer to) [individual name] trading as [business name], which has its principal place of business at [address].

OR

In this disclaimer, "we" means (and "us" and "our" refer to) [*company name*], a company registered in [England and Wales] under registration number [*number*].

OR

In this disclaimer, "we" means (and "us" and "our" refer to) [*business name*], a partnership established under [English law] having its principal place of business at [*address*].

oduct-compliance